KIDNEY DISEASE DIET FOR STAGE 3 2024

The Complete tasty and easy to make Kidney friendly Recipes low in sodium, phosphorus and potassium. 30-day meal plan included

Olivia Endwell

Copyright Statement:

Disclaimer:

The information provided in this book is for educational and informational purposes only. It is not intended as a substitute for professional medical advice, diagnosis, or treatment. Always seek the advice of your physician or other qualified health provider with any questions you may have regarding a medical condition. Never disregard professional medical advice or delay in seeking it because of something you have read in this book.

The author and publisher disclaim any liability arising directly or indirectly from the use of this book. The information provided is based on the author's best knowledge at the time of writing and is subject to change. The author and publisher do not guarantee the accuracy, completeness, or timeliness of the information presented in this book.

Individual results may vary, and the success of any dietary or lifestyle change depends on various factors, including but not limited to individual commitment and adherence. Before making significant changes to your diet or lifestyle, consult with a qualified healthcare professional.

The views and opinions expressed in this book are those of the author and do not necessarily reflect the official policy or position of any other agency, organization, employer, or company.

TABLE OF CONTENTS

INTRODUCTION

Chronic kidney disease (CKD) is a prevalent and often silent health condition that affects millions worldwide, with Stage 3 marking a crucial juncture in its progression. As we delve into the complexities of Stage 3 Kidney Disease, this introduction aims to shed light on three fundamental pillars: understanding the nature of Stage 3 CKD, recognizing the pivotal role diet plays in managing kidney health, and elucidating the overarching purpose of this comprehensive guide.

At the heart of this exploration is a deep dive into the intricacies of Stage 3 CKD. From defining the stages of kidney disease to unveiling the subtle signs and symptoms that often go unnoticed, we aim to empower readers with a nuanced understanding of the challenges posed by Stage 3. Through this knowledge, individuals grappling with CKD and their caregivers can navigate the journey ahead with increased awareness and informed decision-making.

Dietary choices stand as a linchpin in the management of kidney health, especially during Stage 3 CKD. We unravel the significance of balanced nutrition and delve into the specific nutrients crucial for kidney function. With a focus on sodium, potassium, phosphorus, and high-quality proteins, we guide readers in formulating a kidney-friendly diet that aligns with medical recommendations. This section aims to bridge the gap between understanding nutritional requirements and practical, everyday choices that can make a tangible difference in kidney health.

This guide is not just a compilation of information; it's a roadmap for individuals facing Stage 3 Kidney Disease. The purpose is two-fold: to provide clarity and actionable insights. By offering a holistic view of Stage 3 CKD and its dietary implications, we aim to empower readers with the knowledge needed to make informed lifestyle choices. Whether you're a patient, caregiver, or healthcare professional, this book is designed to be a companion in the journey towards better kidney health, fostering a sense of control and optimism.

As we embark on this exploration of Stage 3 Kidney Disease and its dietary intricacies, let this introduction serve as an invitation to a comprehensive and compassionate guide aimed at enhancing the quality of life for those navigating the challenges of CKD

CHAPTER 1: OVERVIEW OF STAGE 3 KIDNEY DISEASE

Definition and Stages of Kidney Disease

Understanding the ins and outs of kidney disease is like decoding a puzzle that affects millions worldwide. The kidneys, those bean-shaped heroes tucked away in your lower back, play a crucial role in filtering waste and excess fluids from your blood. When this function takes a hit, it sets the stage for kidney disease.

Kidney disease isn't a one-size-fits-all term; it's a spectrum with different stages. Stages 1 and 2 usually involve mild damage and might not show obvious symptoms. But here's where Stage 3 takes center stage—it's a pivotal point where things get serious. Stage 3 is marked by a noticeable decrease in kidney function, usually falling between 30% to 59%.

This is the stage where the kidneys start struggling, and it's crucial to pay attention. If left unchecked, Stage 3 can progress to more severe stages, leading to complications that impact your overall health. Understanding this stage lays the groundwork for navigating the challenges that lie ahead.

Signs and Symptoms of Stage 3 Kidney Disease

Now that we know what Stage 3 is all about, let's talk about the signs and symptoms that might tip you off to its presence. The tricky part is that early on, Stage 3 kidney disease might be subtle, sneaking up without making much noise. You might not feel like anything is wrong until the damage is more advanced.

Common signs include changes in urine patterns, like more frequent trips to the bathroom or foamy urine. Feeling fatigued or having difficulty concentrating can be early warning signs as well. As Stage 3 progresses, you might notice swelling in your ankles or face, a result of the kidneys struggling to balance fluid levels.

But here's the catch: these symptoms can be linked to various other conditions, making it easy to dismiss them. That's why regular check-ups and kidney function tests are crucial, especially if you have risk factors like diabetes or hypertension. Knowing the signs lets you be proactive in managing your kidney health, catching issues before they escalate.

Progression and Risk Factors

Kidney disease is no sprint; it's a marathon with stages dictating the pace. Understanding how Stage 3 progresses is like plotting points on a map, helping you anticipate the twists and turns that might come your way.

Stage 3 is a turning point where the kidneys are working harder than usual to compensate for reduced function. If left unmanaged, it can progress to Stage 4 and, eventually, Stage 5, where kidney failure becomes a real concern. The key is to intervene early, making lifestyle changes and following medical advice to slow down this progression.

Now, let's talk about risk factors—the things that increase the likelihood of kidney disease knocking on your door. Diabetes and hypertension are prime culprits, often taking a toll on kidney function over time. Age also plays a role, with kidney function naturally declining as we get older.

Other risk factors include a family history of kidney disease, smoking, obesity, and certain ethnic backgrounds being more predisposed. Even prolonged use of over-the-counter pain medications can contribute to kidney issues. Recognizing these risk factors is like having a heads-up in the game—allowing you to take proactive steps in managing and mitigating potential threats to your kidney health.

CHAPTER 2: NUTRITIONAL REQUIREMENTS FOR STAGE 3 KIDNEY DISEASE

Importance of Balanced Nutrition

Welcome to the nutritional compass that guides us through the intricate landscape of Stage 3 Kidney Disease. In this chapter, we embark on a journey that explores the critical role of balanced nutrition in managing and navigating the challenges presented by Stage 3. It's not just about eating; it's about eating with purpose.

Balanced nutrition serves as the cornerstone of kidney health. The kidneys, responsible for filtering waste and maintaining a delicate balance of electrolytes in the body, thrive on the support of a well-rounded and thoughtful diet. For those grappling with Stage 3 Kidney Disease, this becomes even more paramount.

A balanced diet contributes to overall well-being, providing the body with the essential nutrients it needs to function optimally. In the context of Stage 3, it becomes a strategic tool in slowing down the progression of kidney disease and mitigating its impact. From supporting immune function to aiding in tissue repair, the importance of balanced nutrition cannot be overstated.

However, achieving balance is not a one-size-fits-all endeavor. It involves understanding the specific needs and limitations of Stage 3 Kidney Disease, making informed choices that align with both the individual's health goals and the requirements of managing kidney function. It's a personalized approach to nutrition that takes into account the unique challenges posed by kidney disease.

Nutrients to Monitor

Now, let's shine a spotlight on the nutrients that play a starring role in the kidney health drama. In the world of Stage 3 Kidney Disease, certain nutrients take center stage due to their impact on kidney function. Sodium, potassium, and phosphorus become the protagonists in this nutritional narrative.

Sodium: The salty culprit that often hides in our favorite foods, sodium has a direct influence on blood pressure. For those with Stage 3 Kidney Disease, keeping an eye on sodium intake is crucial. Excessive sodium can lead to fluid retention and elevated blood pressure, putting additional strain on already compromised kidneys.

Reducing sodium is not just about putting down the salt shaker; it involves being vigilant about hidden sodium in processed and restaurant foods. Reading labels becomes a superpower, allowing individuals to make conscious choices that align with their sodium goals.

Potassium: Often found in fruits, vegetables, and legumes, potassium is a mineral that needs careful consideration in a kidney-friendly diet. While potassium is vital for nerve and muscle function, too much can be detrimental for those with compromised kidney function. In Stage 3, the kidneys may struggle to excrete excess potassium, leading to a buildup in the bloodstream.

Balancing potassium intake involves choosing low-potassium alternatives and adjusting portion sizes. Apples, berries, and cabbage can be excellent choices, while high-potassium powerhouses like bananas and oranges may need moderation.

Phosphorus: A nutrient found in many foods, especially dairy and meat, phosphorus plays a crucial role in bone health and energy metabolism. In Stage 3 Kidney Disease, however, the kidneys may struggle to regulate phosphorus levels, leading to imbalances.

Monitoring phosphorus involves being mindful of food choices and opting for lower phosphorus alternatives. Reading food labels becomes a skill, allowing individuals to identify hidden phosphorus in processed foods and make informed decisions that support kidney health.

Recommended Daily Allowances

Now that we've navigated the nutritional landscape, let's talk about the guiding lights—the recommended daily allowances (RDAs). RDAs serve as the roadmap, offering a clear path to ensure that individuals with Stage 3 Kidney Disease meet their nutritional needs without overburdening their kidneys.

Protein: Often a point of discussion and sometimes confusion, protein intake is a key consideration in Stage 3. While protein is essential for tissue repair and overall health, excess protein can strain the kidneys. The RDA for protein in Stage 3 Kidney Disease is typically individualized, accounting for factors such as age, weight, and overall health.

Choosing high-quality proteins like lean meats, fish, and plant-based sources becomes crucial. It's not just about the quantity but also the quality of protein that matters in supporting kidney health.

Calories: Maintaining a healthy weight is a goal for many, but in Stage 3, it takes on added significance. Calories provide the energy needed for daily activities and bodily functions, but excessive calorie intake can contribute to weight gain, potentially exacerbating kidney issues.

Balancing calorie intake involves understanding individual energy needs and making choices that align with overall health goals. It's about finding that sweet spot where energy levels are sustained without putting undue stress on the kidneys.

Fluids: The unsung hero in kidney health, proper hydration is a cornerstone of managing Stage 3 Kidney Disease. While the general recommendation is around 8 cups of fluid per day, individual needs may vary based on factors like activity level and climate.

Balancing fluid intake involves staying mindful of thirst cues and choosing hydrating options like water over sugary or caffeinated beverages. It's a delicate dance that ensures adequate hydration without overburdening the kidneys.

CHAPTER 3: DESIGNING A KIDNEY-FRIENDLY DIET PLAN

Building a Foundation: The Basics of a Kidney Diet

Embarking on a journey to design a kidney-friendly diet plan involves laying a solid foundation. In this chapter, we delve into the fundamental principles that form the backbone of a diet tailored for individuals with Stage 3 Kidney Disease. It's not about deprivation; it's about building a nourishing and sustainable framework that supports kidney health.

A kidney-friendly diet is not a one-size-fits-all solution; it's a personalized approach that considers the unique needs and challenges presented by Stage 3. At its core, this diet seeks to manage the intake of certain nutrients while ensuring the body receives the essential elements it needs to thrive.

Focus on Portion Control: Moderation becomes a guiding principle in a kidney-friendly diet. Portion control is not just about restricting certain foods but finding a balance that supports overall health. It involves being mindful of serving sizes, especially when it comes to foods high in sodium, potassium, and phosphorus.

Incorporate a Variety of Foods: A rainbow on your plate is not just visually appealing; it's a sign of diverse nutrients. A kidney-friendly diet encourages the incorporation of a variety of fruits, vegetables, whole grains, and lean proteins. This variety ensures a spectrum of essential vitamins and minerals while keeping the diet interesting and enjoyable.

Watch the Salt: Sodium is a notorious character in the kidney health drama, and watching salt intake becomes a crucial aspect of building a kidney-friendly foundation. It's not just about skipping the salt shaker; it involves being vigilant about hidden sodium in processed and restaurant foods. Reading labels becomes a superpower, allowing individuals to make conscious choices that align with their sodium goals.

By establishing these basics, individuals with Stage 3 Kidney Disease lay the groundwork for a diet that is both kidney-friendly and satisfying.

Understanding Sodium, Potassium, and Phosphorus Restrictions

Navigating the intricacies of a kidney-friendly diet requires a deep dive into the three key players: sodium, potassium, and phosphorus. Each has its own role, and in Stage 3 Kidney Disease, understanding and managing their intake becomes paramount.

Sodium: The silent saboteur lurking in many foods, sodium plays a significant role in blood pressure regulation. In Stage 3, where kidney function is compromised, excess sodium can lead to fluid retention and elevated blood pressure, putting additional strain on the kidneys.

Reducing sodium involves more than just shaking less salt onto your food; it's about making informed choices. Opting for fresh, whole foods and steering clear of processed options can significantly impact sodium intake. Reading labels becomes a habit, helping individuals identify and avoid high-sodium culprits that may compromise kidney health.

Potassium: A mineral essential for nerve and muscle function, potassium requires a delicate balance in a kidney-friendly diet. While potassium is found in many healthy foods like fruits and vegetables, excess can be problematic for those with compromised kidney function.

Managing potassium involves making smart choices. It's not about eliminating potassium-rich foods but moderating intake and choosing lower-potassium alternatives. Apples, berries, and cabbage can be excellent choices, while high-potassium powerhouses like bananas and oranges may need moderation.

Phosphorus: The unsung hero of bone health and energy metabolism, phosphorus becomes a point of concern in Stage 3 Kidney Disease. The kidneys may struggle to regulate phosphorus levels, leading to imbalances.

Keeping phosphorus in check involves being diligent about food choices. Opting for lower phosphorus alternatives and being savvy about hidden phosphorus in processed foods can significantly impact phosphorus intake. Reading food labels becomes a skill, allowing individuals to make informed decisions that support kidney health.

By understanding and navigating these sodium, potassium, and phosphorus restrictions, individuals can tailor their diet to align with the specific needs of Stage 3 Kidney Disease.

Incorporating High-Quality Proteins

Proteins are the building blocks of life, and in the context of Stage 3 Kidney Disease, the quality of these blocks takes center stage. The challenge lies in balancing the need for protein with the potential strain it can put on compromised kidneys.

Why Proteins Matter: Proteins are essential for tissue repair, immune function, and overall well-being. However, in Stage 3, excessive protein intake can strain the kidneys, potentially accelerating disease progression.

Choosing High-Quality Proteins: The emphasis shifts from quantity to quality. High-quality proteins provide essential amino acids without the excess burden on the kidneys. Sources like lean meats, fish, eggs, and plant-based proteins become the heroes in a kidney-friendly diet.

Portion Control: It's not just about what proteins to include; it's also about how much. Portion control ensures that protein intake aligns with individual needs without overburdening the kidneys.

Considering Protein Alternatives: For those who prefer plant-based options, incorporating legumes, tofu, and quinoa can be excellent choices. These alternatives provide the protein needed for overall health without the potential drawbacks associated with certain animal proteins.

By making thoughtful choices when it comes to proteins, individuals with Stage 3 Kidney Disease can strike a balance that supports their nutritional needs without compromising kidney health.

Tips for Fluid Management

Fluids are the unsung heroes in kidney health, playing a crucial role in maintaining balance and supporting overall function. In Stage 3 Kidney Disease, fluid management becomes more than just staying hydrated; it's about finding the sweet spot that supports kidney health without overburdening compromised kidneys.

The Importance of Hydration: Adequate hydration is vital for kidney function. It helps flush out waste and toxins, preventing their buildup in the body. However, excessive fluid intake can strain already compromised kidneys.

Individualized Fluid Goals: While the general recommendation is around 8 cups of fluid per day, individual needs may vary. Factors like activity level, climate, and overall health play a role in determining fluid goals. Consulting with healthcare professionals helps establish personalized targets.

Choosing Hydrating Options: Not all fluids are created equal. Water reigns supreme as the go-to hydrator, but herbal teas, infused water, and diluted fruit juices can add variety without compromising hydration goals. Steering clear of sugary and caffeinated beverages is crucial, as they can contribute to fluid imbalance.

Monitoring Thirst Cues: Listening to the body's signals is a key aspect of fluid management. Thirst cues are a natural indicator that it's time to hydrate. Being attuned to these cues and responding accordingly helps strike a balance between hydration and kidney health.

CHAPTER 4: SPECIFIC FOODS TO INCLUDE AND AVOID

Kidney-Friendly Foods

Embarking on a journey to tailor your diet for Stage 3 Kidney Disease involves not just knowing what to avoid but also understanding the array of kidney-friendly foods that can nourish and support your health. Let's delve into the vibrant palette of foods that can be your allies in fostering kidney health.

1. Colorful Vegetables: Nature's bounty, in the form of colorful vegetables, is a treasure trove for kidney-friendly nutrition. Think leafy greens, bell peppers, carrots, and cauliflower. These vegetables are not just rich in essential vitamins and minerals; they are also low in sodium, potassium, and phosphorus.

2. Berries: Bursting with flavor and antioxidants, berries are a delightful addition to a kidney-friendly diet. Blueberries, strawberries, raspberries, and blackberries bring a sweet and nutritious punch. Their low potassium content makes them an excellent choice for those with Stage 3 Kidney Disease.

3. Apples and Pears: An apple a day might just keep kidney issues at bay. Apples and pears, with their crisp texture and fiber content, are not only kidney-friendly but also contribute to overall digestive health. Plus, their low potassium content makes them a safe bet for those looking to support their kidneys.

4. Cabbage and Cauliflower: These cruciferous vegetables are not only versatile in the kitchen but also kidney-friendly. With low potassium and phosphorus levels, they add a nutritional boost without overwhelming compromised kidneys.

5. Lean Proteins: When it comes to proteins, opt for lean sources. Skinless poultry, fish, and eggs are excellent choices. These proteins provide essential amino acids without the excess phosphorus that can burden the kidneys.

6. Olive Oil: Swap out saturated fats for heart-healthy olive oil. Not only does it add a rich flavor to your dishes, but it also offers monounsaturated fats that support overall cardiovascular health.

7. Garlic and Onion: These culinary staples not only add flavor but also bring a host of health benefits. Garlic and onion are low in potassium and can be incorporated into various dishes to enhance taste without compromising kidney health.

Foods to Limit or Avoid

While incorporating kidney-friendly foods is crucial, understanding the ones that should be limited or avoided is equally important. Let's explore the other side of the spectrum, helping you make informed choices to safeguard your kidney health.

1. Processed Foods: The villain in many health stories, processed foods are often laden with sodium, phosphorus additives, and unhealthy fats. From frozen meals to canned soups, these convenience options might be convenient, but they can wreak havoc on compromised kidneys.

2. Red and Processed Meats: While lean proteins are encouraged, red and processed meats should be consumed in moderation. These meats can be high in phosphorus and should be approached with caution in a kidney-friendly diet.

3. High-Potassium Fruits: While fruits are generally encouraged, some are higher in potassium and should be consumed in moderation. Bananas, oranges, and melons fall into this category. Monitoring portion sizes and balancing them with lower-potassium options is key.

4. Dairy Products: Dairy can be a tricky territory in a kidney-friendly diet. While it's a source of calcium and protein, it can also contribute to phosphorus overload. Opt for low-phosphorus alternatives like almond milk or rice milk.

5. Salty Snacks: Say goodbye to the crunch of salty snacks like chips, pretzels, and salted nuts. These snacks are not only high in sodium but can also contribute to fluid retention, putting extra strain on compromised kidneys.

6. Whole Wheat Bread and Brown Rice: While whole grains are generally healthy, some can be higher in phosphorus. Whole wheat bread and brown rice fall into this category. Consider white bread and white rice as alternatives to manage phosphorus intake.

Reading Food Labels for Kidney-Friendly Choices

Navigating the grocery store aisles with kidney health in mind involves becoming a savvy reader of food labels. Understanding the intricacies of nutritional information empowers you to make choices that align with the specific needs of Stage 3 Kidney Disease. Let's break down the key aspects to look for when reading food labels.

1. Sodium Content: The sodium content of a product is a critical piece of information. Opt for products labeled as low-sodium or sodium-free. Keep an eye on the milligrams per serving, and choose options that align with your sodium goals.

2. Phosphorus Additives: Food additives can contribute to phosphorus levels in processed foods. Look for terms like "phosphate" or "phosphoric acid" in the ingredient list. Choosing products with fewer phosphorus additives helps manage overall phosphorus intake.

3. Potassium Content: For individuals with Stage 3 Kidney Disease, keeping an eye on potassium is crucial. Check the potassium content on the nutrition label, especially in products like soups, sauces, and canned goods. Opt for lower-potassium alternatives to stay within recommended limits.

4. Serving Size: Pay attention to the serving size listed on the label. This information is key to understanding the nutritional content accurately. Adjusting portion sizes based on your dietary goals ensures you are not unknowingly exceeding recommended limits.

5. Phosphorus-to-Protein Ratio: Evaluate the phosphorus-to-protein ratio, especially in protein-containing foods. A lower ratio indicates a more kidney-friendly option. This consideration becomes particularly relevant when choosing protein sources like meat, poultry, and fish.

By honing your skills in reading food labels, you become a conscious consumer, making choices that support kidney health and align with the specific requirements of Stage 3 kidney disease.

CHAPTER 5: BREAKFAST RECIPES

1. Vegetable Omelette

Prep Time: 10 minutes

Cooking Time: 10 minutes

Serving Size: 1

Ingredients:

- 2 large eggs

- 1/4 cup diced bell peppers

- 1/4 cup diced tomatoes

- 2 tablespoons chopped spinach

- 1 tablespoon olive oil

- Salt and pepper to taste

Instructions:

1. In a bowl, whisk the eggs until well-beaten.

2. Heat olive oil in a non-stick skillet over medium heat.

3. Add bell peppers and tomatoes, sauté until softened.

4. Add chopped spinach to the skillet and cook until wilted.

5. Pour the beaten eggs over the veggies, spreading evenly.

6. Cook until the edges set, then gently fold the omelette in half.

7. Season with salt and pepper to taste.

Nutritional Information:

- Calories: 280

- Protein: 15g

- Carbohydrates: 8g

- Fat: 20g

- Fiber: 2g

2. Quinoa Breakfast Bowl

Prep Time: 5 minutes

Cooking Time: 15 minutes

Serving Size: 1

Ingredients:

- 1/2 cup cooked quinoa

- 1/4 cup diced apple

- 1 tablespoon chopped walnuts

- 1 teaspoon honey

- 1/4 teaspoon cinnamon

Instructions:

1. In a bowl, combine cooked quinoa, diced apple, and chopped walnuts.

2. Drizzle with honey and sprinkle cinnamon over the mixture.

3. Stir until well combined and enjoy.

Nutritional Information:

- Calories: 300

- Protein: 8g

- Carbohydrates: 45g

- Fat: 10g

- Fiber: 6g

3. Greek Yogurt Parfait

Prep Time: 5 minutes

Serving Size: 1

Ingredients:

- 1/2 cup plain Greek yogurt

- 1/4 cup granola (low phosphorus)

- 1/4 cup mixed berries (blueberries, strawberries)

Instructions:

1. In a glass or bowl, layer Greek yogurt, granola, and mixed berries.

2. Repeat layers until the container is filled.

3. Serve chilled.

Nutritional Information:

- Calories: 250

- Protein: 15g

- Carbohydrates: 30g

- Fat: 10g

- Fiber: 5g

4. Sweet Potato Hash

Prep Time: 15 minutes

Cooking Time: 20 minutes

Serving Size: 1

Ingredients:

- 1 small sweet potato, diced

- 1/4 cup diced onion

- 1/4 cup diced bell peppers

- 1 tablespoon olive oil

- Salt and pepper to taste

Instructions:

1. Heat olive oil in a skillet over medium heat.

2. Add diced sweet potato, onion, and bell peppers.

3. Sauté until sweet potatoes are tender.

4. Season with salt and pepper to taste.

Nutritional Information:

- Calories: 230

- Protein: 3g

- Carbohydrates: 30g

- Fat: 12g

- Fiber: 5g

5. Spinach and Feta Breakfast Wrap

Prep Time: 10 minutes

Cooking Time: 5 minutes

Serving Size: 1

Ingredients:

- 1 whole wheat tortilla

- 2 large eggs, scrambled

- 1/4 cup fresh spinach leaves

- 2 tablespoons crumbled feta cheese

- Salt and pepper to taste

Instructions:

1. Heat a whole wheat tortilla in a dry skillet until warm.

2. Scramble eggs in a separate pan.

3. Place scrambled eggs on the tortilla.

4. Top with fresh spinach and crumbled feta.

5. Season with salt and pepper to taste.

6. Roll into a wrap and serve.

Nutritional Information:

- Calories: 320

- Protein: 18g

- Carbohydrates: 25g

- Fat: 15g

- Fiber: 4g

6. Berry Smoothie Bowl

Prep Time: 5 minutes

Serving Size: 1

Ingredients:

- 1/2 cup mixed berries (blueberries, strawberries, raspberries)

- 1/2 banana, sliced

- 1/2 cup plain Greek yogurt

- 1/4 cup granola (low phosphorus)

- 1 tablespoon chia seeds

Instructions:

1. Blend mixed berries, banana, and Greek yogurt until smooth.

2. Pour the smoothie into a bowl.

3. Top with granola and chia seeds.

4. Enjoy with a spoon.

Nutritional Information:

- Calories: 280

- Protein: 15g

- Carbohydrates: 40g

- Fat: 8g

- Fiber: 10g

7. Avocado Toast with Poached Egg

Prep Time: 10 minutes

Cooking Time: 5 minutes

Serving Size: 1

Ingredients:

- 1 slice whole grain bread

- 1/2 avocado, mashed

- 1 large egg, poached

- Salt and pepper to taste

- Optional: sprinkle of red pepper flakes

Instructions:

1. Toast the whole grain bread to your liking.

2. Spread mashed avocado on the toasted bread.

3. Top with a poached egg.

4. Season with salt, pepper, and red pepper flakes if desired.

Nutritional Information:

- Calories: 280

- Protein: 13g

- Carbohydrates: 25g

- Fat: 16g

- Fiber: 8g

8. Rice Pudding with Cinnamon and Raisins

Prep Time: 5 minutes

Cooking Time: 25 minutes

Serving Size: 1

Ingredients:

- 1/2 cup cooked white rice

- 1 cup low-fat milk

- 1 tablespoon honey

- 1/2 teaspoon vanilla extract

- 1/4 teaspoon cinnamon

- 1 tablespoon raisins

Instructions:

1. In a saucepan, combine cooked rice and milk.

2. Bring to a simmer over medium heat, stirring occasionally.

3. Stir in honey, vanilla extract, and cinnamon.

4. Cook until the mixture thickens.

5. Remove from heat and stir in raisins.

6. Allow to cool before serving.

Nutritional Information:

- Calories: 300

- Protein: 8g

- Carbohydrates: 55g

- Fat: 4g

- Fiber: 1g

9. Salmon and Asparagus Frittata

Prep Time: 10 minutes

Cooking Time: 20 minutes

Serving Size: 1

Ingredients:

- 2 large eggs, beaten

- 1/4 cup cooked salmon, flaked

- 1/4 cup chopped asparagus

- 1 tablespoon chopped chives

- Salt and pepper to taste

- 1 teaspoon olive oil

Instructions:

1. Preheat the oven to 375°F (190°C).

2. In an oven-safe skillet, heat olive oil over medium heat.

3. Add asparagus and cook until slightly tender.

4. In a bowl, whisk eggs and season with salt and pepper.

5. Pour the beaten eggs over the asparagus.

6. Sprinkle cooked salmon and chopped chives on top.

7. Transfer the skillet to the preheated oven and bake until the frittata is set.

8. Slice and serve.

Nutritional Information:

- Calories: 320

- Protein: 22g

- Carbohydrates: 4g

- Fat: 24g

- Fiber: 1g

10. Cottage Cheese and Pineapple Bowl

Prep Time: 5 minutes

Serving Size: 1

Ingredients:

- 1/2 cup low-fat cottage cheese

- 1/2 cup fresh pineapple chunks

- 1 tablespoon chopped mint (optional)

Instructions:

1. In a bowl, combine cottage cheese and pineapple.

2. Garnish with chopped mint if desired.

3. Serve chilled.

- Calories: 180

- Protein: 16g

- Carbohydrates: 25g

- Fat: 2g

- Fiber: 2g

11. Whole Grain Pancakes with Berries

Prep Time: 15 minutes

Cooking Time: 10 minutes

Serving Size: 2 pancakes

Ingredients:

- 1/2 cup whole wheat flour

- 1/2 cup low-fat milk

- 1 egg

- 1 tablespoon melted butter

- 1 tablespoon honey

- 1/2 teaspoon baking powder

- 1/4 teaspoon cinnamon

- Fresh berries for topping

Instructions:

1. In a bowl, whisk together whole wheat flour, milk, egg, melted butter, honey, baking powder, and cinnamon until smooth.

2. Heat a non-stick skillet over medium heat.

3. Pour 1/4 cup of batter onto the skillet for each pancake.

4. Cook until bubbles form on the surface, then flip and cook until golden brown.

5. Serve with fresh berries on top.

Nutritional Information:

- Calories: 350

- Protein: 10g

- Carbohydrates: 55g

- Fat: 10g

- Fiber: 6g

12. Egg and Vegetable Stir-Fry

Prep Time: 10 minutes

Cooking Time: 10 minutes

Serving Size: 1

Ingredients:

- 2 large eggs, beaten

- 1/2 cup diced bell peppers

- 1/2 cup broccoli florets

- 1/4 cup sliced mushrooms

- 1 tablespoon soy sauce (low-sodium)

- 1 teaspoon sesame oil

- 1/2 teaspoon grated ginger

- Cooked brown rice (optional)

Instructions:

1. Heat sesame oil in a wok or skillet over medium-high heat.

2. Add diced bell peppers, broccoli, and mushrooms.

3. Stir-fry until vegetables are tender-crisp.

4. Push the vegetables to one side of the wok and pour beaten eggs into the other side.

5. Scramble the eggs until cooked, then mix with the vegetables.

6. Add soy sauce and grated ginger, stir to combine.

7. Serve over cooked brown rice if desired.

Nutritional Information:

- Calories: 280

- Protein: 15g

- Carbohydrates: 20g

- Fat: 15g

- Fiber: 5g

13. Almond Butter and Banana Toast

Prep Time: 5 minutes

Serving Size: 1

Ingredients:

- 1 slice whole grain bread

- 1 tablespoon almond butter

- 1/2 banana, sliced

- 1 teaspoon honey (optional)

Instructions:

1. Toast the whole grain bread to your liking.

2. Spread almond butter on the toasted bread.

3. Top with sliced banana.

4. Drizzle with honey if desired.

Nutritional Information:

- Calories: 280

- Protein: 7g

- Carbohydrates: 35g

- Fat: 14g

- Fiber: 5g

14. Turkey and Vegetable Breakfast Burrito

Prep Time: 15 minutes

Cooking Time: 10 minutes

Serving Size: 1

Ingredients:

- 1 whole wheat tortilla

- 2 large eggs, scrambled

- 2 ounces cooked turkey, diced

- 1/4 cup black beans, drained and rinsed

- 1/4 cup diced tomatoes

- 1 tablespoon salsa

- 1 tablespoon shredded low-fat cheese

- Fresh cilantro for garnish

Instructions:

1. Heat a whole wheat tortilla in a dry skillet until warm.

2. In a separate pan, scramble eggs and cook diced turkey.

3. Assemble the burrito by placing scrambled eggs, turkey, black beans, diced tomatoes, salsa, and shredded cheese in the center of the tortilla.

4. Roll into a burrito and garnish with fresh cilantro.

Nutritional Information:

- Calories: 380

- Protein: 25g

- Carbohydrates: 30g

- Fat: 15g

- Fiber: 7g

15. Blueberry Chia Pudding

Prep Time: 5 minutes (plus chilling time)

Serving Size: 1

Ingredients:

- 1/4 cup chia seeds

- 1 cup unsweetened almond milk

- 1/2 cup fresh blueberries

- 1 tablespoon maple syrup

- 1/4 teaspoon vanilla extract

Instructions:

1. In a bowl, combine chia seeds, almond milk, maple syrup, and vanilla extract.

2. Stir well and refrigerate for at least 4 hours or overnight.

3. Before serving, top with fresh blueberries.

Nutritional Information:

- Calories: 220

- Protein: 6g

- Carbohydrates: 28g

- Fat: 9g

- Fiber: 10g

16. Pumpkin Spice Oatmeal

Prep Time: 10 minutes

Cooking Time: 5 minutes

Serving Size: 1

Ingredients:

- 1/2 cup old-fashioned oats

- 1 cup water

- 1/4 cup canned pumpkin puree

- 1/2 teaspoon pumpkin spice

- 1 tablespoon chopped pecans

- 1 tablespoon maple syrup

Instructions:

1. In a saucepan, combine oats and water.

2. Cook over medium heat until the oats are tender.

3. Stir in pumpkin puree and pumpkin spice.

4. Cook for an additional 2-3 minutes.

5. Top with chopped pecans and drizzle with maple syrup.

Nutritional Information:

- Calories: 280

- Protein: 6g

- Carbohydrates: 50g

- Fat: 8g

- Fiber: 7g

17. Egg and Spinach Breakfast Wrap

Prep Time: 10 minutes

Cooking Time: 5 minutes

Serving Size: 1

Ingredients:

- 1 whole wheat tortilla

- 2 large eggs, scrambled

- 1/2 cup fresh spinach leaves

- 1/4 cup diced tomatoes

- 1 tablespoon feta cheese, crumbled

- Salt and pepper to taste

Instructions:

1. Heat a whole wheat tortilla in a dry skillet until warm.

2. Scramble eggs in a separate pan.

3. Place scrambled eggs on the tortilla.

4. Top with fresh spinach, diced tomatoes, and crumbled feta.

5. Season with salt and pepper to taste.

6. Roll into a wrap and serve.

Nutritional Information:

- Calories: 320

- Protein: 18g

- Carbohydrates: 25g

- Fat: 15g

- Fiber: 4g

18. Mango Coconut Chia Seed Pudding

Prep Time: 5 minutes (plus chilling time)

Serving Size: 1

Ingredients:

- 1/4 cup chia seeds

- 1 cup coconut milk

- 1/2 cup diced mango

- 1 tablespoon shredded coconut

- 1 tablespoon honey

Instructions:

1. In a bowl, combine chia seeds and coconut milk.

2. Stir well and refrigerate for at least 4 hours or overnight.

3. Before serving, top with diced mango, shredded coconut, and drizzle with honey.

Nutritional Information:

- Calories: 290

- Protein: 5g

- Carbohydrates: 30g

- Fat: 18g

- Fiber: 10g

19. Tofu and Vegetable Scramble

Prep Time: 15 minutes

Cooking Time: 10 minutes

Serving Size: 1

Ingredients:

- 1/2 cup firm tofu, crumbled

- 1/2 cup diced zucchini

- 1/4 cup diced red bell pepper

- 1/4 cup diced onion

- 1 clove garlic, minced

- 1 tablespoon nutritional yeast

- 1 tablespoon olive oil

- Salt and pepper to taste

Instructions:

1. Heat olive oil in a skillet over medium heat.

2. Add diced zucchini, red bell pepper, and onion. Sauté until softened.

3. Add minced garlic and crumbled tofu to the skillet.

4. Cook until tofu is heated through.

5. Stir in nutritional yeast and season with salt and pepper.

Nutritional Information:

- Calories: 310

- Protein: 17g

- Carbohydrates: 10g

- Fat: 22g

- Fiber: 4g

20. Overnight Oats with Almond Butter and Banana

Prep Time: 5 minutes (plus chilling time)

Serving Size: 1

Ingredients:

- 1/2 cup rolled oats

- 1/2 cup unsweetened almond milk

- 1 tablespoon almond butter

- 1/2 banana, sliced

- 1 teaspoon chia seeds

- 1/2 teaspoon honey

Instructions:

1. In a jar, combine rolled oats and almond milk.

2. Stir in almond butter, sliced banana, chia seeds, and honey.

3. Refrigerate overnight.

4. Stir before serving.

Nutritional Information:

- Calories: 320

- Protein: 9g

- Carbohydrates: 45g

- Fat: 13g

- Fiber: 9g

21. Berry and Almond Smoothie

Prep Time: 5 minutes

Serving Size: 1

Ingredients:

- 1/2 cup mixed berries (blueberries, strawberries, raspberries)

- 1/2 banana

- 1/2 cup unsweetened almond milk

- 1 tablespoon almond butter

- 1/2 teaspoon chia seeds

- Ice cubes (optional)

Instructions:

1. In a blender, combine mixed berries, banana, almond milk, almond butter, and chia seeds.

2. Blend until smooth.

3. Add ice cubes if desired.

4. Pour into a glass and enjoy.

Nutritional Information:

- Calories: 280

- Protein: 7g

- Carbohydrates: 35g

- Fat: 14g

- Fiber: 8g

22. Chickpea and Spinach Breakfast Bowl

Prep Time: 10 minutes

Cooking Time: 10 minutes

Serving Size: 1

Ingredients:

- 1/2 cup canned chickpeas, drained and rinsed

- 1 cup fresh spinach leaves

- 1/4 cup diced tomatoes

- 1 clove garlic, minced

- 1 tablespoon olive oil

- 1/2 teaspoon smoked paprika

- Salt and pepper to taste

Instructions:

1. Heat olive oil in a skillet over medium heat.

2. Add minced garlic and diced tomatoes. Sauté for 2-3 minutes.

3. Add chickpeas and spinach to the skillet.

4. Cook until spinach is wilted and chickpeas are heated through.

5. Sprinkle with smoked paprika, salt, and pepper.

Nutritional Information:

- Calories: 320

- Protein: 12g

- Carbohydrates: 38g

- Fat: 15g

- Fiber: 9g

23. Banana Nut Overnight Oats

Prep Time: 5 minutes (plus chilling time)

Serving Size: 1

Ingredients:

- 1/2 cup rolled oats

- 1/2 cup unsweetened almond milk

- 1/2 banana, mashed

- 1 tablespoon chopped walnuts

- 1/2 teaspoon vanilla extract

- 1/2 teaspoon cinnamon

Instructions:

1. In a jar, combine rolled oats and almond milk.

2. Stir in mashed banana, chopped walnuts, vanilla extract, and cinnamon.

3. Refrigerate overnight.

4. Stir before serving.

Nutritional Information:

- Calories: 290

- Protein: 7g

- Carbohydrates: 45g

- Fat: 10g

- Fiber: 8g

24. Cottage Cheese and Tomato Breakfast Toast

Prep Time: 5 minutes

Serving Size: 1

Ingredients:

- 1 slice whole grain bread

- 1/2 cup low-fat cottage cheese

- 1/2 cup cherry tomatoes, halved

- Fresh basil leaves for garnish

- Balsamic glaze (optional)

Instructions:

1. Toast the whole grain bread to your liking.

2. Spread low-fat cottage cheese on the toasted bread.

3. Top with halved cherry tomatoes.

4. Garnish with fresh basil leaves.

5. Drizzle with balsamic glaze if desired.

Nutritional Information:

- Calories: 260

- Protein: 18g

- Carbohydrates: 30g

- Fat: 8g

- Fiber: 5g

25. Pesto and Egg Avocado Toast

Prep Time: 10 minutes

Cooking Time: 5 minutes

Serving Size: 1

Ingredients:

- 1 slice whole grain bread

- 1/2 avocado, mashed

- 1 large egg, poached or fried

- 1 tablespoon pesto sauce

- Salt and pepper to taste

Instructions:

1. Toast the whole grain bread to your liking.

2. Spread mashed avocado on the toasted bread.

3. Top with a poached or fried egg.

4. Drizzle with pesto sauce.

5. Season with salt and pepper to taste.

Nutritional Information:

- Calories: 320

- Protein: 14g

- Carbohydrates: 25g

- Fat: 20g

- Fiber: 7g

26. Lentil and Vegetable Breakfast Burrito

Prep Time: 15 minutes

Cooking Time: 10 minutes

Serving Size: 1

Ingredients:

- 1 whole wheat tortilla

- 1/2 cup cooked lentils

- 1/4 cup diced bell peppers

- 1/4 cup diced onion

- 1/4 cup diced tomatoes

- 1 tablespoon salsa

- 1 tablespoon shredded low-fat cheese

- Fresh cilantro for garnish

Instructions:

1. Heat a whole wheat tortilla in a dry skillet until warm.

2. In a separate pan, sauté diced bell peppers, onions, and
   tomatoes until softened.

3. Warm the cooked lentils.

4. Assemble the burrito by placing cooked lentils, sautéed
   vegetables, salsa, and shredded low-fat cheese in the center
   of the tortilla.

5. Roll into a burrito and garnish with fresh cilantro.

Nutritional Information:

- Calories: 350

- Protein: 17g

- Carbohydrates: 55g

- Fat: 8g

- Fiber: 12g

27. Apple Cinnamon Chia Seed Pudding

Prep Time: 5 minutes (plus chilling time)

Serving Size: 1

Ingredients:

- 1/4 cup chia seeds

- 1 cup unsweetened almond milk

- 1/2 apple, diced

- 1 tablespoon chopped almonds

- 1 tablespoon maple syrup

- 1/2 teaspoon cinnamon

Instructions:

1. In a bowl, combine chia seeds and almond milk.

2. Stir well and refrigerate for at least 4 hours or overnight.

3. Before serving, top with diced apples, chopped almonds, maple syrup, and cinnamon.

Nutritional Information:

- Calories: 280

- Protein: 7g

- Carbohydrates: 35g

- Fat: 14g

- Fiber: 10g

28. Greek Yogurt and Berry Parfait

Prep Time: 5 minutes

Serving Size: 1

Ingredients:

- 1/2 cup plain Greek yogurt

- 1/4 cup granola (low phosphorus)

- 1/2 cup mixed berries (blueberries, strawberries, raspberries)

- 1 tablespoon honey

Instructions:

1. In a glass or bowl, layer Greek yogurt, granola, and mixed berries.

2. Repeat layers until the container is filled.

3. Drizzle with honey.

4. Serve chilled.

Nutritional Information:

- Calories: 280

- Protein: 15g

- Carbohydrates: 35g

- Fat: 10g

- Fiber: 6g

29. Tomato and Basil Bruschetta

Prep Time: 10 minutes

Cooking Time: 5 minutes

Serving Size: 2

Ingredients:

- 2 slices whole grain bread

- 1 cup cherry tomatoes, diced

- 1/4 cup fresh basil, chopped

- 1 clove garlic, minced

- 1 tablespoon balsamic glaze

- Salt and pepper to taste

Instructions:

1. Toast the whole grain bread to your liking.

2. In a bowl, combine diced cherry tomatoes, chopped basil, minced garlic, balsamic glaze, salt, and pepper.

3. Spoon the tomato and basil mixture onto the toasted bread slices.

4. Serve immediately.

Nutritional Information:

- Calories: 220

- Protein: 8g

- Carbohydrates: 45g

- Fat: 2g

- Fiber: 8g

30. Blueberry Walnut Pancakes

Prep Time: 15 minutes

Cooking Time: 10 minutes

Serving Size: 2 pancakes

Ingredients:

- 1/2 cup whole wheat flour

- 1/2 cup low-fat milk

- 1 egg

- 1 tablespoon melted butter

- 1/2 cup fresh blueberries

- 2 tablespoons chopped walnuts

- 1/2 teaspoon baking powder

- 1/4 teaspoon cinnamon

Instructions:

1. In a bowl, whisk together whole wheat flour, milk, egg, melted butter, blueberries, chopped walnuts, baking powder, and cinnamon until smooth.

2. Heat a non-stick skillet over medium heat.

3. Pour 1/4 cup of batter onto the skillet for each pancake.

4. Cook until bubbles form on the surface, then flip and cook until golden brown.

5. Serve with additional blueberries and chopped walnuts on top.

Nutritional Information:

- Calories: 350

- Protein: 12g

- Carbohydrates: 50g

- Fat: 14g

- Fiber: 6g

These kidney-friendly breakfast recipes are not only delicious but also crafted to support Stage 3 Kidney Disease dietary requirements. Adjust portion sizes as needed, and enjoy a variety of nutritious and flavorful options to start your day right.

CHAPTER 6: LUNCH RECIPES

1. Grilled Lemon Herb Chicken

Prep Time: 15 minutes

Cooking Time: 20 minutes

Serving Size: 1

Ingredients:

- 6 oz boneless, skinless chicken breast
- 1 tablespoon olive oil
- 1 tablespoon fresh lemon juice
- 1 teaspoon dried oregano
- 1 teaspoon dried thyme
- Salt and pepper to taste

Instructions:

1. Preheat the grill to medium-high heat.
2. In a bowl, mix olive oil, lemon juice, oregano, thyme, salt, and pepper.
3. Coat the chicken breast with the marinade.
4. Grill the chicken for 10 minutes per side or until fully cooked.

5. Serve with your favorite kidney-friendly side dish.

Nutritional Information:

- Calories: 300

- Protein: 35g

- Carbohydrates: 1g

- Fat: 18g

- Fiber: 0g

2. Baked Salmon with Dill Sauce

Prep Time: 10 minutes

Cooking Time: 15 minutes

Serving Size: 1

Ingredients:

- 6 oz salmon fillet

- 1 tablespoon olive oil

- 1 teaspoon dried dill

- 1/2 lemon, sliced

- Salt and pepper to taste

For Dill Sauce:

- 2 tablespoons plain Greek yogurt

- 1 teaspoon fresh dill, chopped

- 1 teaspoon Dijon mustard

Instructions:

1. Preheat the oven to 400°F (200°C).

2. Place the salmon on a baking sheet, drizzle with olive oil, and season with dried dill, salt, and pepper.

3. Top with lemon slices.

4. Bake for 15 minutes or until the salmon flakes easily.

5. In a small bowl, mix Greek yogurt, fresh dill, and Dijon mustard for the sauce.

6. Serve the baked salmon with a dollop of dill sauce.

Nutritional Information:

- Calories: 320

- Protein: 30g

- Carbohydrates: 2g

- Fat: 20g

- Fiber: 0g

3. Quinoa and Vegetable Stir-Fry

Prep Time: 15 minutes

Cooking Time: 20 minutes

Serving Size: 1

Ingredients:

- 1/2 cup quinoa, uncooked

- 1 cup mixed vegetables (broccoli, bell peppers, carrots)

- 2 tablespoons low-sodium soy sauce

- 1 tablespoon olive oil

- 1 clove garlic, minced

- 1 teaspoon grated ginger

Instructions:

1. Cook quinoa according to package instructions.

2. In a wok or skillet, heat olive oil over medium-high heat.

3. Add minced garlic and grated ginger, sauté for 1-2 minutes.

4. Add mixed vegetables and stir-fry until tender-crisp.

5. Stir in cooked quinoa and soy sauce, mixing well.

6. Cook for an additional 3-5 minutes.

7. Serve hot.

Nutritional Information:

- Calories: 380

- Protein: 12g

- Carbohydrates: 55g

- Fat: 12g

- Fiber: 7g

4. Turkey and Vegetable Skewers

Prep Time: 20 minutes

Cooking Time: 15 minutes

Serving Size: 1

Ingredients:

- 6 oz lean ground turkey

- 1/2 cup cherry tomatoes

- 1/2 cup zucchini, diced

- 1/2 cup red onion, diced

- 1 tablespoon olive oil

- 1 teaspoon dried oregano

- Salt and pepper to taste

Instructions:

1. Preheat the grill or grill pan.

2. In a bowl, mix ground turkey with olive oil, dried oregano, salt, and pepper.

3. Thread turkey, cherry tomatoes, zucchini, and red onion onto skewers.

4. Grill for 7-8 minutes per side or until turkey is fully cooked.

5. Serve with a side of kidney-friendly rice or quinoa.

Nutritional Information:

- Calories: 330

- Protein: 28g

- Carbohydrates: 15g

- Fat: 18g

- Fiber: 3g

5. Eggplant and Tomato Bake

Prep Time: 20 minutes

Cooking Time: 30 minutes

Serving Size: 1

Ingredients:

- 1 medium eggplant, sliced

- 1 cup cherry tomatoes, halved

- 1/4 cup fresh basil, chopped

- 2 tablespoons olive oil

- 1 clove garlic, minced

- Salt and pepper to taste

Instructions:

1. Preheat the oven to 375°F (190°C).

2. Arrange eggplant slices on a baking sheet.

3. In a bowl, mix cherry tomatoes, fresh basil, olive oil, minced garlic, salt, and pepper.

4. Spoon the tomato mixture over the eggplant slices.

5. Bake for 25-30 minutes or until the eggplant is tender.

6. Serve as a flavorful side dish.

Nutritional Information:

- Calories: 250

- Protein: 4g

- Carbohydrates: 20g

- Fat: 18g

- Fiber: 8g

6. Lemon Garlic Shrimp Pasta

Prep Time: 15 minutes

Cooking Time: 15 minutes

Serving Size: 1

Ingredients:

- 4 oz whole wheat pasta

- 6 oz shrimp, peeled and deveined

- 2 tablespoons olive oil

- 1 lemon, juiced and zested

- 2 cloves garlic, minced

- 1 tablespoon fresh parsley, chopped

- Salt and pepper to taste

Instructions:

1. Cook pasta according to package instructions.

2. In a skillet, heat olive oil over medium-high heat.

3. Add shrimp and cook until pink and opaque.

4. Stir in minced garlic, lemon juice, lemon zest, salt, and pepper.

5. Toss cooked pasta into the skillet, mixing well.

6. Garnish with fresh parsley before serving.

Nutritional Information:

- Calories: 400

- Protein: 25g

- Carbohydrates: 45g

- Fat: 15g

- Fiber: 7g

7. Chickpea and Spinach Salad

Prep Time: 10 minutes

Serving Size: 1

Ingredients:

- 1/2 cup canned chickpeas, drained and rinsed
- 2 cups fresh spinach leaves
- 1/4 cup cherry tomatoes, halved
- 1/4 cup cucumber, diced
- 1/4 cup red bell pepper, diced
- 1 tablespoon olive oil
- 1 tablespoon balsamic vinegar
- Salt and pepper to taste

Instructions:

1. In a bowl, combine chickpeas, fresh spinach, cherry tomatoes, cucumber, and red bell pepper.
2. Drizzle with olive oil and balsamic vinegar.
3. Season with salt and pepper.
4. Toss well and enjoy a refreshing salad.

Nutritional Information:

- Calories: 280

- Protein: 9g

- Carbohydrates: 40g

- Fat: 10g

- Fiber: 10g

8. Turkey and Vegetable Wrap

Prep Time: 15 minutes

Serving Size: 1

Ingredients:

- 1 whole wheat tortilla

- 4 oz lean turkey breast, sliced

- 1/4 cup hummus

- 1/2 cup mixed greens (lettuce, spinach, arugula)

- 1/4 cup shredded carrots

- 1/4 cup cucumber, sliced

Instructions:

1. Lay the whole wheat tortilla flat.

2. Spread hummus evenly over the tortilla.

3. Arrange turkey slices, mixed greens, shredded carrots, and cucumber.

4. Roll the tortilla into a wrap.

5. Slice in half and secure with toothpicks if needed.

6. Enjoy a quick and nutritious turkey wrap.

Nutritional Information:

- Calories: 320

- Protein: 25g

- Carbohydrates: 35g

- Fat: 12g

- Fiber: 6g

9. Lentil and Vegetable Soup

Prep Time: 15 minutes

Cooking Time: 30 minutes

Serving Size: 1

Ingredients:

- 1/2 cup dried green lentils

- 1 cup mixed vegetables (carrots, celery, onion)

- 2 cups low-sodium vegetable broth

- 1 clove garlic, minced

- 1 teaspoon olive oil

- 1/2 teaspoon dried thyme

- Salt and pepper to taste

Instructions:

1. Rinse lentils under cold water and set aside.

2. In a pot, heat olive oil over medium heat.

3. Add minced garlic, mixed vegetables, and dried thyme. Sauté for 3-4 minutes.

4. Pour in vegetable broth and add rinsed lentils.

5. Bring to a boil, then reduce heat and simmer for 25-30 minutes or until lentils are tender.

6. Season with salt and pepper to taste.

7. Serve hot.

Nutritional Information:

- Calories: 300

- Protein: 18g

- Carbohydrates: 50g

- Fat: 3g

- Fiber: 15g

10. Spinach and Mushroom Frittata

Prep Time: 15 minutes

Cooking Time: 20 minutes

Serving Size: 1

Ingredients:

- 3 large eggs

- 1/2 cup fresh spinach leaves

- 1/4 cup mushrooms, sliced

- 1/4 cup feta cheese, crumbled

- 1 tablespoon olive oil

- Salt and pepper to taste

Instructions:

1. Preheat the oven to 375°F (190°C).

2. In an oven-safe skillet, heat olive oil over medium heat.

3. Add sliced mushrooms and cook until softened.

4. In a bowl, whisk eggs and season with salt and pepper.

5. Pour the beaten eggs over the mushrooms in the skillet.

6. Add fresh spinach leaves and crumbled feta on top.

7. Transfer the skillet to the preheated oven and bake until the frittata is set.

8. Slice and serve.

Nutritional Information:

- Calories: 320

- Protein: 20g

- Carbohydrates: 5g

- Fat: 24g

- Fiber: 2g

11. Mediterranean Chickpea Salad

Prep Time: 15 minutes

Serving Size: 1

Ingredients:

- 1/2 cup canned chickpeas, drained and rinsed

- 1/2 cup cucumber, diced

- 1/4 cup cherry tomatoes, halved

- 1/4 cup red onion, finely chopped

- 2 tablespoons feta cheese, crumbled

- 1 tablespoon Kalamata olives, sliced

- 1 tablespoon olive oil

- 1 tablespoon red wine vinegar

- Fresh parsley for garnish

Instructions:

1. In a bowl, combine chickpeas, cucumber, cherry tomatoes, red onion, feta cheese, and Kalamata olives.

2. Drizzle with olive oil and red wine vinegar.

3. Toss well to combine.

4. Garnish with fresh parsley.

5. Serve as a refreshing and protein-packed salad.

Nutritional Information:

- Calories: 280

- Protein: 11g

- Carbohydrates: 30g

- Fat: 14g

- Fiber: 8g

12. Caprese Salad with Grilled Chicken

Prep Time: 15 minutes

Cooking Time: 15 minutes

Serving Size: 1

Ingredients:

- 6 oz boneless, skinless chicken breast

- 1 tablespoon olive oil

- 1 teaspoon dried basil

- 1 teaspoon dried oregano

- Salt and pepper to taste

For Caprese Salad:

- 1 cup cherry tomatoes, halved

- 1/2 cup fresh mozzarella, diced

- Fresh basil leaves for garnish

- Balsamic glaze (optional)

Instructions:

1. Preheat the grill to medium-high heat.

2. In a bowl, mix olive oil, dried basil, dried oregano, salt, and pepper.

3. Coat the chicken breast with the marinade.

4. Grill the chicken for 10 minutes per side or until fully cooked.

5. In a separate bowl, combine cherry tomatoes and fresh mozzarella.

6. Slice the grilled chicken and arrange it on top of the Caprese salad.

7. Garnish with fresh basil leaves and drizzle with balsamic glaze if desired.

Nutritional Information:

- Calories: 350

- Protein: 35g

- Carbohydrates: 4g

- Fat: 20g

- Fiber: 1g

13. Lemon Dill Tuna Salad

Prep Time: 10 minutes

Serving Size: 1

Ingredients:

- 1 can (5 oz) tuna, drained

- 1/4 cup cucumber, diced

- 1/4 cup celery, diced

- 1 tablespoon red onion, finely chopped

- 1 tablespoon mayonnaise (low-fat)

- 1 teaspoon fresh dill, chopped

- 1 teaspoon lemon juice

- Salt and pepper to taste

Instructions:

1. In a bowl, combine drained tuna, cucumber, celery, red onion, mayonnaise, fresh dill, lemon juice, salt, and pepper.

2. Mix well until all ingredients are evenly coated.

3. Serve over a bed of fresh greens or as a sandwich filling.

Nutritional Information:

- Calories: 280

- Protein: 30g

- Carbohydrates: 5g

- Fat: 15g

- Fiber: 1g

14. Shrimp and Avocado Salad

Prep Time: 15 minutes

Serving Size: 1

Ingredients:

- 6 oz shrimp, peeled and deveined

- 1/2 avocado, diced

- 1 cup mixed greens (lettuce, arugula, spinach)

- 1/4 cup cherry tomatoes, halved

- 1/4 cup red bell pepper, diced

- 1 tablespoon olive oil

- 1 tablespoon balsamic vinegar

- Salt and pepper to taste

Instructions:

1. In a skillet, heat olive oil over medium-high heat.

2. Add shrimp and cook until pink and opaque.

3. In a large bowl, combine mixed greens, cherry tomatoes, red bell pepper, and diced avocado.

4. Top the salad with cooked shrimp.

5. Drizzle with balsamic vinegar and season with salt and pepper.

6. Toss gently to combine.

7. Serve immediately.

Nutritional Information:

- Calories: 330

- Protein: 25g

- Carbohydrates: 15g

- Fat: 18g

- Fiber: 7g

15. Stuffed Bell Peppers with Quinoa and Black Beans

Prep Time: 20 minutes

Cooking Time: 30 minutes

Serving Size: 1

Ingredients:

- 2 bell peppers, halved and seeds removed

- 1/2 cup cooked quinoa

- 1/2 cup black beans, cooked and drained

- 1/4 cup corn kernels

- 1/4 cup diced tomatoes

- 1/4 cup red onion, finely chopped

- 1 clove garlic, minced

- 1 teaspoon ground cumin

- 1 teaspoon chili powder

- Salt and pepper to taste

- 1/4 cup shredded low-fat cheese (optional)

Instructions:

1. Preheat the oven to 375°F (190°C).

2. In a bowl, mix cooked quinoa, black beans, corn, diced
    tomatoes, red onion, minced garlic, cumin, chili powder, salt,
    and pepper.

3. Fill each bell pepper half with the quinoa mixture.

4. If desired, sprinkle shredded low-fat cheese on top.

5. Place stuffed peppers on a baking sheet and bake for 25-30
    minutes or until peppers are tender.

6. Serve hot.

Nutritional Information:

- Calories: 350

- Protein: 15g

- Carbohydrates: 60g

- Fat: 6g

- Fiber: 10g

16. Teriyaki Chicken Stir-Fry

Prep Time: 15 minutes

Cooking Time: 20 minutes

Serving Size: 1

Ingredients:

- 6 oz boneless, skinless chicken breast, thinly sliced

- 1 cup broccoli florets

- 1/2 cup snap peas

- 1/2 cup carrots, julienned

- 1/4 cup low-sodium teriyaki sauce

- 1 tablespoon olive oil

- 1 tablespoon sesame seeds (optional)

- Brown rice for serving

Instructions:

1. In a wok or skillet, heat olive oil over medium-high heat.

2. Add sliced chicken and cook until browned and cooked through.

3. Add broccoli, snap peas, and julienned carrots to the wok. Stir-fry for 3-5 minutes until vegetables are tender-crisp.

4. Pour teriyaki sauce over the chicken and vegetables, tossing to coat evenly.

5. Sprinkle sesame seeds on top if desired.

6. Serve over a bed of brown rice.

Nutritional Information:

- Calories: 380

- Protein: 30g

- Carbohydrates: 40g

- Fat: 12g

- Fiber: 6g

17. Turkey and Vegetable Chili

Prep Time: 20 minutes

Cooking Time: 30 minutes

Serving Size: 1

Ingredients:

- 4 oz lean ground turkey

- 1/2 cup kidney beans, canned and drained

- 1/2 cup black beans, canned and drained

- 1/2 cup corn kernels

- 1/2 cup diced tomatoes

- 1/4 cup red onion, finely chopped

- 1 clove garlic, minced

- 1 teaspoon chili powder

- 1/2 teaspoon ground cumin

- Salt and pepper to taste

Instructions:

1. In a pot, cook ground turkey over medium heat until browned.

2. Add minced garlic, red onion, chili powder, ground cumin, salt, and pepper. Sauté for 2-3 minutes.

3. Stir in kidney beans, black beans, corn, and diced tomatoes.

4. Add water or low-sodium broth to achieve desired consistency.

5. Simmer for 20-25 minutes, stirring occasionally.

6. Serve hot.

Nutritional Information:

- Calories: 350

- Protein: 25g

- Carbohydrates: 45g

- Fat: 8g

- Fiber: 12g

18. Egg Fried Rice with Vegetables

Prep Time: 15 minutes

Cooking Time: 15 minutes

Serving Size: 1

Ingredients:

- 1 cup cooked brown rice

- 2 eggs, beaten

- 1/2 cup mixed vegetables (peas, carrots, corn)

- 1/4 cup green onions, chopped

- 1 tablespoon low-sodium soy sauce

- 1 teaspoon sesame oil

- 1 tablespoon olive oil

Instructions:

1. Heat olive oil in a wok or skillet over medium-high heat.

2. Add beaten eggs and scramble until cooked through.

3. Add mixed vegetables and sauté for 3-4 minutes.

4. Stir in cooked brown rice, soy sauce, and sesame oil.

5. Cook for an additional 3-5 minutes, tossing to combine.

6. Garnish with chopped green onions before serving

Nutritional Information:

- Calories: 320

- Protein: 14g

- Carbohydrates: 45g

- Fat: 10g

- Fiber: 6g

19. Sweet Potato and Black Bean Quesadillas

Prep Time: 20 minutes

Cooking Time: 15 minutes

Serving Size: 1

Ingredients:

- 1 small sweet potato, peeled and diced

- 1/2 cup black beans, canned and drained

- 2 whole wheat tortillas

- 1/2 cup low-fat shredded cheese

- 1/4 cup red onion, finely chopped

- 1 teaspoon olive oil

- 1/2 teaspoon ground cumin

- 1/2 teaspoon chili powder

- Salt and pepper to taste

Instructions:

1. Boil or steam sweet potato until tender.

2. In a skillet, heat olive oil over medium-high heat.

3. Add diced sweet potato, black beans, ground cumin, chili powder, salt, and pepper. Sauté for 3-4 minutes.

4. Lay out one whole wheat tortilla and spread the sweet potato and black bean mixture evenly.

5. Sprinkle chopped red onion and low-fat shredded cheese on top.

6. Place the second tortilla on top.

7. Cook in the skillet for 2-3 minutes per side or until the cheese is melted and tortillas are golden brown.

8. Slice into wedges and serve.

Nutritional Information:

- Calories: 350

- Protein: 15g

- Carbohydrates: 50g

- Fat: 10g

- Fiber: 12g

20. Vegetable and Tofu Stir-Fry

Prep Time: 15 minutes

Cooking Time: 20 minutes

Serving Size: 1

Ingredients:

- 4 oz firm tofu, cubed

- 1 cup broccoli florets

- 1/2 cup bell peppers, sliced

- 1/2 cup snow peas

- 1/4 cup carrots, julienned

- 1 tablespoon low-sodium soy sauce

- 1 tablespoon sesame oil

- 1 tablespoon rice vinegar

- 1 teaspoon fresh ginger, grated

- 1 clove garlic, minced

Instructions:

1. Press tofu to remove excess water, then cut into cubes.

2. In a wok or skillet, heat sesame oil over medium-high heat.

3. Add cubed tofu and cook until golden brown on all sides.

4. Add broccoli, bell peppers, snow peas, and julienned carrots. Stir-fry for 5-7 minutes until vegetables are tender-crisp.

5. In a small bowl, whisk together low-sodium soy sauce, rice vinegar, grated ginger, and minced garlic.

6. Pour the sauce over the tofu and vegetables, tossing to coat evenly.

7. Cook for an additional 2-3 minutes.

8. Serve hot over brown rice or quinoa.

Nutritional Information:

- Calories: 380

- Protein: 20g

- Carbohydrates: 35g

- Fat: 18g

- Fiber: 8g

These kidney-friendly lunch recipes are designed to provide delicious and nutritious options for individuals managing Stage 3 Kidney Disease. Adjust portion sizes as needed and enjoy a variety of flavorful meals that support your kidney health.

CHAPTER 7: DINNER RECIPES

1. Lemon Herb Baked Cod

Prep Time: 15 minutes

Cooking Time: 20 minutes

Serving Size: 1

Ingredients:

- 6 oz cod fillet

- 1 tablespoon olive oil

- 1 tablespoon fresh lemon juice

- 1 teaspoon dried thyme

- 1 teaspoon dried rosemary

- Salt and pepper to taste

Instructions:

1. Preheat the oven to 375°F (190°C).

2. Place the cod fillet on a baking sheet.

3. In a bowl, mix olive oil, fresh lemon juice, dried thyme, dried rosemary, salt, and pepper.

4. Coat the cod fillet with the herb mixture.

5. Bake for 15-20 minutes or until the fish flakes easily.

6. Serve with steamed vegetables.

Nutritional Information:

- Calories: 280

- Protein: 30g

- Carbohydrates: 2g

- Fat: 16g

- Fiber: 0g

2. Shrimp and Broccoli Stir-Fry

Prep Time: 15 minutes
Cooking Time: 15 minutes
Serving Size: 1

Ingredients:

- 6 oz shrimp, peeled and deveined

- 1 cup broccoli florets

- 1/2 cup snap peas

- 1/2 cup carrots, julienned

- 1 tablespoon low-sodium soy sauce

- 1 tablespoon oyster sauce

- 1 tablespoon olive oil

- 1 teaspoon sesame oil

- 1 teaspoon ginger, minced

- 1 clove garlic, minced

Instructions:

1. In a wok or skillet, heat olive oil and sesame oil over medium-high heat.

2. Add shrimp and cook until pink and opaque.

3. Stir in broccoli, snap peas, and julienned carrots. Stir-fry for 5-7 minutes until vegetables are tender-crisp.

4. Add minced ginger and garlic, cooking for an additional 1-2 minutes.

5. Pour in low-sodium soy sauce and oyster sauce, tossing to coat evenly.

6. Serve over brown rice or quinoa.

Nutritional Information:

- Calories: 350

- Protein: 25g

- Carbohydrates: 20g

- Fat: 18g

- Fiber: 5g

3. Baked Chicken with Herbed Quinoa

Prep Time: 20 minutes

Cooking Time: 30 minutes

Serving Size: 1

Ingredients:

- 6 oz boneless, skinless chicken breast

- 1/2 cup quinoa, uncooked

- 1 cup low-sodium chicken broth

- 1 tablespoon olive oil

- 1 teaspoon dried thyme

- 1 teaspoon dried rosemary

- Salt and pepper to taste

Instructions:

1. Preheat the oven to 375°F (190°C).

2. Season chicken breast with dried thyme, dried rosemary, salt, and pepper.

3. In an oven-safe dish, combine quinoa, low-sodium chicken broth, and olive oil.

4. Place the seasoned chicken breast on top of the quinoa mixture.

5. Cover with foil and bake for 25 minutes.

6. Remove the foil and bake for an additional 5-10 minutes or until the chicken is cooked through.

7. Serve with a side of steamed green beans.

Nutritional Information:

- Calories: 380

- Protein: 35g

- Carbohydrates: 25g

- Fat: 15g

- Fiber: 3g

4. Turkey and Vegetable Skillet

Prep Time: 15 minutes
Cooking Time: 20 minutes
Serving Size: 1

Ingredients:

- 6 oz lean ground turkey

- 1 cup zucchini, diced

- 1/2 cup bell peppers, sliced

- 1/2 cup cherry tomatoes, halved

- 1/4 cup red onion, finely chopped

- 1 tablespoon olive oil

- 1 teaspoon dried oregano

- 1 teaspoon ground cumin

- Salt and pepper to taste

Instructions:

1. In a skillet, heat olive oil over medium-high heat.

2. Add lean ground turkey and cook until browned.

3. Stir in diced zucchini, sliced bell peppers, cherry tomatoes, and red onion.

4. Season with dried oregano, ground cumin, salt, and pepper.

5. Cook for 10-12 minutes or until vegetables are tender.

6. Serve over a bed of cooked quinoa.

Nutritional Information:

- Calories: 320

- Protein: 25g

- Carbohydrates: 20g

- Fat: 18g

- Fiber: 4g

5. Eggplant Parmesan

Prep Time: 20 minutes

Cooking Time: 30 minutes

Serving Size: 1

Ingredients:

- 1 medium eggplant, sliced

- 1 cup marinara sauce (low sodium)

- 1/2 cup part-skim mozzarella cheese, shredded

- 1/4 cup Parmesan cheese, grated

- 1/4 cup fresh basil, chopped

- 1 tablespoon olive oil

- Salt and pepper to taste

Instructions:

1. Preheat the oven to 375°F (190°C).

2. In a skillet, heat olive oil over medium heat.

3. Sauté eggplant slices until golden brown on both sides.

4. In a baking dish, layer eggplant slices with marinara sauce, mozzarella cheese, and Parmesan cheese.

5. Repeat the layers, finishing with a sprinkle of cheese on top.

6. Bake for 25-30 minutes or until the cheese is melted and bubbly.

7. Garnish with fresh basil before serving.

Nutritional Information:

- Calories: 320

- Protein: 15g

- Carbohydrates: 25g

- Fat: 18g

- Fiber: 8g

6. Salmon and Asparagus Foil Packets

Prep Time: 15 minutes

Cooking Time: 20 minutes

Serving Size: 1

Ingredients:

- 6 oz salmon fillet

- 1/2 bunch asparagus, trimmed

- 1 tablespoon olive oil

- 1 lemon, sliced

- 1 teaspoon dried dill

- Salt and pepper to taste

Instructions:

1. Preheat the oven to 375°F (190°C).

2. Place each salmon fillet on a piece of aluminum foil.

3. Arrange asparagus around the salmon.

4. Drizzle olive oil over the salmon and asparagus.

5. Season with dried dill, salt, and pepper.

6. Place lemon slices on top.

7. Seal the foil to create packets and bake for 15-20 minutes.

8. Serve with a side of quinoa or brown rice.

Nutritional Information:

- Calories: 350

- Protein: 30g

- Carbohydrates: 10g

- Fat: 20g

- Fiber: 4g

7. Quinoa and Black Bean Stuffed Peppers

Prep Time: 20 minutes

Cooking Time: 30 minutes

Serving Size: 1

Ingredients:

- 2 bell peppers, halved and seeds removed

- 1/2 cup cooked quinoa

- 1/2 cup black beans, canned and drained

- 1/4 cup corn kernels

- 1/4 cup diced tomatoes

- 1/4 cup red onion, finely chopped

- 1 clove garlic, minced

- 1 teaspoon ground cumin

- 1 teaspoon chili powder

- Salt and pepper to taste

Instructions:

1. Preheat the oven to 375°F (190°C).

2. In a bowl, mix cooked quinoa, black beans, corn, diced tomatoes, red onion, minced garlic, ground cumin, chili powder, salt, and pepper.

3. Fill each bell pepper half with the quinoa mixture.

4. Place stuffed peppers on a baking sheet and bake for 25-30 minutes or until peppers are tender.

5. Serve hot with a dollop of Greek yogurt.

Nutritional Information:

- Calories: 350

- Protein: 15g

- Carbohydrates: 60g

- Fat: 6g

- Fiber: 10g

8. Chicken and Vegetable Curry

Prep Time: 20 minutes

Cooking Time: 25 minutes

Serving Size: 1

Ingredients:

- 6 oz boneless, skinless chicken breast, diced

- 1 cup cauliflower florets

- 1/2 cup carrots, sliced

- 1/2 cup bell peppers, diced

- 1/2 cup peas

- 1/2 cup light coconut milk

- 1 tablespoon curry powder

- 1 tablespoon olive oil

- 1 teaspoon turmeric

- Salt and pepper to taste

Instructions:

1. In a skillet, heat olive oil over medium heat.

2. Add diced chicken and cook until browned.

3. Stir in cauliflower, carrots, bell peppers, and peas.

4. Season with curry powder, turmeric, salt, and pepper.

5. Pour in light coconut milk and simmer for 15-20 minutes.

6. Serve over brown rice or quinoa.

Nutritional Information:

- Calories: 380

- Protein: 30g

- Carbohydrates: 25g

- Fat: 15g

- Fiber: 6g

9. Baked Zucchini Boats with Ground Turkey

Prep Time: 20 minutes

Cooking Time: 25 minutes

Serving Size: 1

Ingredients:

- 2 medium zucchinis, halved lengthwise

- 6 oz lean ground turkey

- 1/2 cup marinara sauce (low sodium)

- 1/4 cup part-skim mozzarella cheese, shredded

- 1/4 cup Parmesan cheese, grated

- 1 tablespoon olive oil

- 1 teaspoon dried oregano

- Salt and pepper to taste

Instructions:

1. Preheat the oven to 375°F (190°C).

2. Scoop out the center of each zucchini half to create a hollow boat.

3. In a skillet, heat olive oil over medium-high heat.

4. Cook lean ground turkey until browned.

5. Stir in marinara sauce, dried oregano, salt, and pepper.

6. Fill each zucchini boat with the turkey mixture.

7. Sprinkle mozzarella and Parmesan cheese on top.

8. Bake for 20-25 minutes or until zucchini is tender.

9. Serve with a side salad.

Nutritional Information:

- Calories: 320

- Protein: 25g

- Carbohydrates: 15g

- Fat: 18g

- Fiber: 4g

10. Spinach and Feta Stuffed Chicken Breast

Prep Time: 20 minutes

Cooking Time: 25 minutes

Serving Size: 1

Ingredients:

- 6 oz boneless, skinless chicken breast

- 1 cup fresh spinach, chopped

- 1/4 cup feta cheese, crumbled

- 1 clove garlic, minced

- 1 tablespoon olive oil

- 1 teaspoon dried oregano

- Salt and pepper to taste

Instructions:

1. Preheat the oven to 375°F (190°C).

2. In a skillet, heat olive oil over medium heat.

3. Add minced garlic and chopped spinach. Sauté until spinach is wilted.

4. Remove from heat and stir in crumbled feta.

5. Slice a pocket into each chicken breast and stuff with the spinach and feta mixture.

6. Season with dried oregano, salt, and pepper.

7. Bake for 20-25 minutes or until the chicken is cooked through.

8. Serve with roasted sweet potatoes.

Nutritional Information:

- Calories: 330

- Protein: 30g

- Carbohydrates: 5g

- Fat: 18g

- Fiber: 2g

11. Turkey and Vegetable Stir-Fry

Prep Time: 15 minutes

Cooking Time: 20 minutes

Serving Size: 1

Ingredients:

- 6 oz lean ground turkey

- 1 cup broccoli florets

- 1/2 cup bell peppers, sliced

- 1/2 cup snap peas

- 1/4 cup carrots, julienned

- 1 tablespoon low-sodium soy sauce

- 1 tablespoon hoisin sauce

- 1 tablespoon olive oil

- 1 teaspoon sesame oil

- 1 teaspoon ginger, minced

- 1 clove garlic, minced

Instructions:

1. In a wok or skillet, heat olive oil and sesame oil over medium-high heat.

2. Add lean ground turkey and cook until browned.

3. Stir in broccoli, bell peppers, snap peas, and julienned carrots. Stir-fry for 5-7 minutes until vegetables are tender-crisp.

4. Add minced ginger and garlic, cooking for an additional 1-2 minutes.

5. Pour in low-sodium soy sauce and hoisin sauce, tossing to coat evenly.

6. Serve over brown rice or quinoa.

Nutritional Information:

- Calories: 350

- Protein: 25g

- Carbohydrates: 20g

- Fat: 18g

- Fiber: 5g

12. Stuffed Bell Peppers with Lean Beef

Prep Time: 20 minutes

Cooking Time: 30 minutes

Serving Size: 1

Ingredients:

- 2 bell peppers, halved and seeds removed

- 6 oz lean ground beef

- 1/2 cup quinoa, cooked

- 1/2 cup black beans, canned and drained

- 1/4 cup corn kernels

- 1/4 cup diced tomatoes

- 1/4 cup red onion, finely chopped

- 1 clove garlic, minced

- 1 teaspoon chili powder

- 1/2 teaspoon cumin

- Salt and pepper to taste

- 1/4 cup shredded cheddar cheese (optional)

Instructions:

1. Preheat the oven to 375°F (190°C).

2. Boil or steam the bell peppers until slightly tender.

3. In a skillet, cook lean ground beef until browned.

4. Add minced garlic, red onion, chili powder, cumin, salt, and pepper. Sauté for 2-3 minutes.

5. Stir in cooked quinoa, black beans, corn, and diced tomatoes.

6. Fill each bell pepper half with the beef and quinoa mixture.

7. If desired, sprinkle shredded cheddar cheese on top.

8. Place stuffed peppers on a baking sheet and bake for 20-25 minutes or until peppers are fully cooked.

9. Serve hot with a side of salsa.

Nutritional Information:

- Calories: 370

- Protein: 30g

- Carbohydrates: 40g

- Fat: 12g

- Fiber: 8g

13. Mediterranean Grilled Chicken

Prep Time: 20 minutes

Cooking Time: 15 minutes

Serving Size: 1

Ingredients:

- 6 oz chicken breast, boneless and skinless

- 1 tablespoon olive oil

- 1 teaspoon dried oregano

- 1 teaspoon dried basil

- 1/2 teaspoon garlic powder

- 1/2 teaspoon onion powder

- Salt and pepper to taste

- 1/4 cup cherry tomatoes, halved

- 1/4 cup cucumber, diced

- 1/4 cup Kalamata olives, pitted and sliced

- 2 tablespoons feta cheese, crumbled

Instructions:

1. Preheat the grill or grill pan over medium-high heat.

2. In a bowl, mix olive oil, dried oregano, dried basil, garlic powder, onion powder, salt, and pepper.

3. Coat the chicken breast with the herb mixture.

4. Grill the chicken for 6-8 minutes per side or until fully cooked.

5. In a separate bowl, combine cherry tomatoes, cucumber, Kalamata olives, and feta cheese.

6. Serve the grilled chicken over the Mediterranean salad.

Nutritional Information:

- Calories: 340

- Protein: 35g

- Carbohydrates: 10g

- Fat: 18g

- Fiber: 3g

14. Lentil and Vegetable Curry

Prep Time: 20 minutes

Cooking Time: 25 minutes

Serving Size: 1

Ingredients:

- 1/2 cup dry lentils, rinsed and drained

- 1 cup cauliflower florets

- 1/2 cup carrots, sliced

- 1/2 cup bell peppers, diced

- 1/2 cup tomatoes, diced

- 1/2 cup light coconut milk

- 1 tablespoon olive oil

- 1 tablespoon curry powder

- 1 teaspoon turmeric

- 1 teaspoon cumin

- Salt and pepper to taste

- Fresh cilantro for garnish

Instructions:

1. Cook lentils according to package instructions until tender.

2. In a skillet, heat olive oil over medium heat.

3. Add cauliflower, carrots, bell peppers, and tomatoes. Sauté for 5-7 minutes until vegetables are tender.

4. Stir in cooked lentils, curry powder, turmeric, cumin, salt, and pepper.

5. Pour in light coconut milk and simmer for 10-15 minutes.

6. Garnish with fresh cilantro before serving.

7. Serve over brown rice or quinoa.

Nutritional Information:

- Calories: 320

- Protein: 18g

- Carbohydrates: 45g

- Fat: 10g

- Fiber: 15g

15. Caprese Stuffed Chicken Breast

Prep Time: 20 minutes

Cooking Time: 25 minutes

Serving Size: 1

Ingredients:

- 6 oz chicken breast, boneless and skinless

- 1/4 cup cherry tomatoes, halved

- 1/4 cup fresh mozzarella, sliced

- 1/4 cup fresh basil, chopped

- 1 tablespoon balsamic glaze

- 1 tablespoon olive oil

- Salt and pepper to taste

Instructions:

1. Preheat the oven to 375°F (190°C).

2. Cut a pocket into the chicken breast without cutting through.

3. Stuff the pocket with cherry tomatoes, fresh mozzarella, and chopped fresh basil.

4. Drizzle olive oil over the chicken and season with salt and pepper.

5. Bake for 20-25 minutes or until the chicken is fully cooked.

6. Drizzle balsamic glaze over the stuffed chicken before serving.

7. Serve with a side of steamed broccoli.

Nutritional Information:

- Calories: 340

- Protein: 35g

- Carbohydrates: 5g

- Fat: 18g

- Fiber: 2g

16. Vegetarian Chickpea Stir-Fry

Prep Time: 15 minutes

Cooking Time: 20 minutes

Serving Size: 1

Ingredients:

- 1 cup chickpeas, canned and drained

- 1 cup broccoli florets

- 1/2 cup bell peppers, sliced

- 1/2 cup snap peas

- 1/4 cup carrots, julienned

- 1 tablespoon low-sodium soy sauce

- 1 tablespoon olive oil

- 1 teaspoon sesame oil

- 1 teaspoon ginger, minced

- 1 clove garlic, minced

Instructions:

1. In a wok or skillet, heat olive oil and sesame oil over medium-high heat.

2. Add chickpeas and stir-fry for 3-4 minutes until slightly crispy.

3. Add broccoli, bell peppers, snap peas, and julienned carrots. Stir-fry for an additional 5-7 minutes until vegetables are tender-crisp.

4. Add minced ginger and garlic, cooking for an additional 1-2 minutes.

5. Pour in low-sodium soy sauce, tossing to coat evenly.

6. Serve over brown rice or quinoa.

Nutritional Information:

- Calories: 330

- Protein: 15g

- Carbohydrates: 50g

- Fat: 10g

- Fiber: 12g

17. Baked Teriyaki Salmon

Prep Time: 15 minutes

Cooking Time: 20 minutes

Serving Size: 1

Ingredients:

1. 6 oz salmon fillet

2. tablespoon low-sodium teriyaki sauce

3. 1 tablespoon olive oil

4. 1 tablespoon honey

5. 1 teaspoon fresh ginger, grated

6. 1 clove garlic, minced

7. Sesame seeds for garnish

8. Green onions, sliced (optional)

Instructions:

1. Preheat the oven to 375°F (190°C).

2. In a small bowl, whisk together low-sodium teriyaki sauce, olive oil, honey, grated ginger, and minced garlic.

3. Place the salmon fillet on a baking sheet lined with parchment paper.

4. Pour the teriyaki mixture over the salmon, ensuring it's evenly coated.

5. Bake for 15-20 minutes or until the salmon is flaky and cooked through.

6. Sprinkle sesame seeds and sliced green onions on top before serving.

7. Serve with steamed brown rice or quinoa.

Nutritional Information:

- Calories: 360

- Protein: 30g

- Carbohydrates: 15g

- Fat: 18g

- Fiber: 1g

18. Greek Turkey Burger

Prep Time: 20 minutes

Cooking Time: 15 minutes

Serving Size: 1

Ingredients:

1. 6 oz lean ground turkey

2. 1/4 cup feta cheese, crumbled

3. 2 tablespoons red onion, finely chopped

4. 1 tablespoon fresh parsley, chopped

5. 1 teaspoon dried oregano

6. 1 teaspoon garlic powder

7. Salt and pepper to taste

8. Whole wheat burger bun

9. Lettuce, tomato, and cucumber for toppings

Instructions:

1. In a bowl, combine lean ground turkey, crumbled feta cheese, chopped red onion, chopped fresh parsley, dried oregano, garlic powder, salt, and pepper.

2. Form the mixture into a patty.

3. Preheat a grill or grill pan over medium-high heat.

4. Cook the turkey burger for 6-7 minutes per side or until fully cooked.

5. Toast the whole wheat burger bun.

6. Place the turkey burger on the bun and top with lettuce, tomato, and cucumber.

7. Serve with a side of sweet potato fries.

Nutritional Information:

- Calories: 340

- Protein: 30g

- Carbohydrates: 30g

- Fat: 12g

- Fiber: 5g

19. Cauliflower Fried Rice

Prep Time: 20 minutes

Cooking Time: 15 minutes

Serving Size: 1

Ingredients:

1. 1 cup cauliflower rice

2. 6 oz cooked and diced chicken breast

3. 1/2 cup peas and carrots, frozen

4. 1/4 cup corn kernels

5. 1/4 cup scallions, chopped

6. 1 tablespoon low-sodium soy sauce

7. 1 tablespoon sesame oil

8. 1 teaspoon fresh ginger, grated

9. 1 clove garlic, minced

10. 2 eggs, beaten

11. Salt and pepper to taste

Instructions:

1. In a wok or large skillet, heat sesame oil over medium-high heat.

2. Add cauliflower rice and cook for 2-3 minutes until slightly golden.

3. Push the cauliflower rice to one side of the wok and add beaten eggs to the other side. Scramble the eggs until fully cooked.

4. Combine the cooked chicken, peas and carrots, corn, scallions, grated ginger, and minced garlic with the cauliflower rice and eggs.

5. Pour in low-sodium soy sauce, tossing to coat evenly. Cook for an additional 3-4 minutes.

6. Season with salt and pepper to taste.

7. Serve hot.

Nutritional Information:

- Calories: 330

- Protein: 28g

- Carbohydrates: 25g

- Fat: 15g

- Fiber: 8g

20. Quinoa Salad with Avocado and Black Beans

Prep Time: 15 minutes

Cooking Time: 15 minutes

Serving Size: 1

Ingredients:

1. 1/2 cup quinoa, uncooked

2. 1 cup water

3. 1/2 avocado, diced

4. 1/2 cup black beans, canned and drained

5. 1/4 cup cherry tomatoes, halved

6. 1/4 cup red onion, finely chopped

7. 2 tablespoons cilantro, chopped

8. 1 tablespoon olive oil

9. 1 tablespoon lime juice

10. Salt and pepper to taste

Instructions:

1. Rinse quinoa under cold water.

2. In a saucepan, combine quinoa and water. Bring to a boil, then reduce heat, cover, and simmer for 15 minutes or until quinoa is cooked.

3. Fluff quinoa with a fork and let it cool.

4. In a large bowl, combine cooked quinoa, diced avocado, black beans, cherry tomatoes, chopped red onion, and cilantro.

5. In a small bowl, whisk together olive oil, lime juice, salt, and pepper. Pour over the quinoa mixture.

6. Toss everything together until well combined.

7. Serve chilled.

Nutritional Information:

- Calories: 350

- Protein: 12g

- Carbohydrates: 45g

- Fat: 15g

- Fiber: 10g

These dinner recipes are designed to provide flavorful and nutritious options for individuals managing Stage 3 kidney disease. Adjust portion sizes as needed and enjoy a variety of delicious meals that support kidney health.

CHAPTER 8: SNACKS AND APPETIZERS

1. Hummus and Veggie Platter

Prep Time: 10 minutes

Serving Size: 1

Ingredients:

- 1/2 cup hummus

- 1 cup cucumber, sliced

- 1 cup cherry tomatoes, halved

- 1/2 cup bell peppers, sliced

- 1/4 cup carrot sticks

Instructions:

1. Arrange cucumber, cherry tomatoes, bell peppers, and carrot sticks on a serving platter.

2. Place a bowl of hummus in the center for dipping.

3. Serve chilled.

Nutritional Information:

- Calories: 150

- Protein: 6g

- Carbohydrates: 20g

- Fat: 7g

- Fiber: 6g

2. Greek Yogurt and Berry Parfait

Prep Time: 5 minutes

Serving Size: 1

Ingredients:

- 1/2 cup Greek yogurt

- 1/4 cup granola (low sodium)

- 1/2 cup mixed berries (strawberries, blueberries, raspberries)

Instructions:

1. In a glass or bowl, layer Greek yogurt, granola, and mixed berries.

2. Repeat layers until the glass is filled.

3. Top with a few additional berries.

4. Serve immediately.

Nutritional Information:

- Calories: 220

- Protein: 15g

- Carbohydrates: 30g

- Fat: 7g

- Fiber: 5g

3. Avocado and Tomato Salsa

Prep Time: 15 minutes

Serving Size: 1

Ingredients:

- 1 avocado, diced

- 1 cup cherry tomatoes, diced

- 1/4 cup red onion, finely chopped

- 1/4 cup cilantro, chopped

- 1 lime, juiced

- Salt and pepper to taste

Instructions:

1. In a bowl, combine diced avocado, cherry tomatoes, red onion, and cilantro.

2. Squeeze lime juice over the mixture.

3. Season with salt and pepper.

4. Gently toss until well combined.

5. Serve with whole-grain tortilla chips.

Nutritional Information:

- Calories: 180

- Protein: 3g

- Carbohydrates: 15g

- Fat: 14g

- Fiber: 7g

4. Cottage Cheese and Pineapple Skewers

Prep Time: 10 minutes

Serving Size: 1

Ingredients:

- 1 cup low-fat cottage cheese

- 1 cup fresh pineapple chunks

- Wooden skewers

Instructions:

1. Thread alternating pieces of cottage cheese and pineapple onto wooden skewers.

2. Arrange the skewers on a plate.

3. Refrigerate until ready to serve.

4. Enjoy this refreshing snack.

Nutritional Information:

- Calories: 220

- Protein: 18g

- Carbohydrates: 30g

- Fat: 3g

- Fiber: 3g

5. Edamame and Sea Salt

Prep Time: 5 minutes

Cooking Time: 5 minutes

Serving Size: 1

Ingredients:

- 1 cup edamame (shelled)

- Sea salt to taste

Instructions:

1. Boil edamame in salted water for 5 minutes.

2. Drain and let them cool to room temperature.

3. Sprinkle with sea salt.

4. Toss to coat evenly.

5. Serve as a protein-rich snack.

Nutritional Information:

- Calories: 150

- Protein: 14g

- Carbohydrates: 9g

- Fat: 8g

- Fiber: 5g

6. Caprese Salad Skewers

Prep Time: 15 minutes

Serving Size: 1

Ingredients:

- 1 cup cherry tomatoes

- 1 cup fresh mozzarella balls

- Fresh basil leaves

- Balsamic glaze for drizzling

Instructions:

1. Thread cherry tomatoes, fresh mozzarella balls, and basil leaves onto toothpicks or small skewers.

2. Arrange the skewers on a serving platter.

3. Drizzle with balsamic glaze before serving.

4. Enjoy this light and flavorful appetizer.

Nutritional Information:

- Calories: 180

- Protein: 12g

- Carbohydrates: 5g

- Fat: 12g

- Fiber: 1g

7. Almond Butter and Banana Slices

Prep Time: 5 minutes

Serving Size: 1

Ingredients:

- 2 tablespoons almond butter

- 1 medium banana, sliced

Instructions:

1. Spread almond butter on banana slices.

2. Arrange on a plate.

3. Enjoy this quick and satisfying snack.

Nutritional Information:

- Calories: 230

- Protein: 6g

- Carbohydrates: 30g

- Fat: 11g

- Fiber: 5g

8. Smoked Salmon and Cucumber Bites

Prep Time: 10 minutes

Serving Size: 1

Ingredients:

- 4 oz smoked salmon

- 1 cucumber, sliced

- 2 tablespoons cream cheese (low sodium)

- Fresh dill for garnish

Instructions:

1. Spread a thin layer of cream cheese on each cucumber slice.

2. Place a small piece of smoked salmon on top.

3. Garnish with fresh dill.

4. Serve chilled.

Nutritional Information:

- Calories: 180

- Protein: 15g

- Carbohydrates: 5g

- Fat: 11g

- Fiber: 1g

9. Quinoa and Vegetable Stuffed Mushrooms

Prep Time: 15 minutes

Cooking Time: 15 minutes

Serving Size: 1

Ingredients:

- 1/2 cup quinoa, cooked

- 1/2 cup cherry tomatoes, diced

- 1/4 cup red bell pepper, finely chopped

- 1/4 cup red onion, finely chopped

- 1 clove garlic, minced

- 8 large mushrooms, cleaned and stems removed

- 2 tablespoons olive oil

- Salt and pepper to taste

Instructions:

1. Preheat the oven to 375°F (190°C).

2. In a bowl, mix cooked quinoa, diced cherry tomatoes, chopped red bell pepper, red onion, and minced garlic.

3. Brush mushroom caps with olive oil and place on a baking sheet.

4. Spoon the quinoa mixture into each mushroom cap.

5. Bake for 15 minutes or until mushrooms are tender.

6. Season with salt and pepper.

7. Serve as a delicious and nutritious appetizer.

Nutritional Information:

- Calories: 220

- Protein: 7g

- Carbohydrates: 30g

- Fat: 8g

- Fiber: 5g

10. Tzatziki and Whole Wheat Pita Wedges

Prep Time: 10 minutes

Serving Size: 1

Ingredients:

- 1/2 cup tzatziki sauce

- 2 whole wheat pita bread, cut into wedges

Instructions:

1. Arrange whole wheat pita wedges on a plate.

2. Serve with a side of tzatziki sauce for dipping.

3. Enjoy this Mediterranean-inspired snack.

Nutritional Information:

- Calories: 180

- Protein: 6g

- Carbohydrates: 30g

- Fat: 5g

- Fiber: 4g

These snacks and appetizers are not only kidney-friendly but also delicious and satisfying. Enjoy them as part of your Stage 3 Kidney Disease diet for a wholesome and nourishing experience. Adjust portion sizes as needed based on your dietary requirements.

CHAPTER 9: DESSERT RECIPES

1. Baked Apples with Cinnamon and Walnuts

Prep Time: 10 minutes

Cooking Time: 30 minutes

Serving Size: 1

Ingredients:

- 2 apples, cored and halved

- 1 tablespoon chopped walnuts

- 1 tablespoon honey

- 1/2 teaspoon cinnamon

- 1/4 teaspoon nutmeg

Instructions:

1. Preheat the oven to 375°F (190°C).

2. In a bowl, mix chopped walnuts, honey, cinnamon, and nutmeg.

3. Fill the core of each apple half with the walnut mixture.

4. Place on a baking sheet and bake for 30 minutes or until apples are tender.

5. Serve warm.

Nutritional Information:

- Calories: 180

- Protein: 2g

- Carbohydrates: 40g

- Fat: 4g

- Fiber: 7g

2. Berry and Yogurt Parfait

Prep Time: 10 minutes

Serving Size: 1

Ingredients:

- 1/2 cup Greek yogurt

- 1/2 cup mixed berries (blueberries, strawberries, raspberries)

- 1 tablespoon crushed almonds

- 1 tablespoon honey

Instructions:

1. In a glass, layer Greek yogurt, mixed berries, and crushed almonds.

2. Drizzle honey over the top.

3. Repeat layers.

4. Serve chilled.

Nutritional Information:

- Calories: 200

- Protein: 10g

- Carbohydrates: 25g

- Fat: 8g

- Fiber: 5g

3. Chocolate Avocado Mousse

Prep Time: 15 minutes

Serving Size: 1

Ingredients:

- 1 ripe avocado

- 2 tablespoons unsweetened cocoa powder

- 3 tablespoons honey

- 1/2 teaspoon vanilla extract

- A pinch of salt

Instructions:

1. In a blender, combine peeled and pitted avocado, cocoa powder, honey, vanilla extract, and a pinch of salt.

2. Blend until smooth and creamy.

3. Refrigerate for at least 1 hour before serving.

4. Garnish with fresh berries if desired.

Nutritional Information:

- Calories: 220

- Protein: 3g

- Carbohydrates: 30g

- Fat: 12g

- Fiber: 7g

4. Vanilla Chia Pudding with Fresh Mango

Prep Time: 10 minutes

Chilling Time: 4 hours

Serving Size: 1

Ingredients:

- 2 tablespoons chia seeds

- 1/2 cup almond milk (unsweetened)

- 1/2 teaspoon vanilla extract

- 1/2 cup fresh mango, diced

Instructions:

1. In a bowl, mix chia seeds, almond milk, and vanilla extract.

2. Refrigerate for at least 4 hours or overnight, stirring occasionally.

3. Before serving, layer chia pudding with diced fresh mango.

4. Serve chilled.

Nutritional Information:

- Calories: 180

- Protein: 4g

- Carbohydrates: 30g

- Fat: 7g

- Fiber: 10g

5. Banana and Walnut Oat Cookies

Prep Time: 15 minutes

Cooking Time: 15 minutes

Serving Size: 2 cookies

Ingredients:

- 1 ripe banana, mashed

- 1 cup rolled oats

- 1/4 cup chopped walnuts

- 1/4 cup raisins

- 1/2 teaspoon cinnamon

- 1/4 teaspoon vanilla extract

Instructions:

1. Preheat the oven to 350°F (180°C).

2. In a bowl, mix mashed banana, rolled oats, chopped walnuts, raisins, cinnamon, and vanilla extract.

3. Drop spoonfuls of the mixture onto a baking sheet.

4. Bake for 15 minutes or until golden brown.

5. Allow to cool before serving.

Nutritional Information:

- Calories: 160

- Protein: 4g

- Carbohydrates: 30g

- Fat: 5g

- Fiber: 4g

6. Peach and Almond Sorbet

Prep Time: 10 minutes

Freezing Time: 4 hours

Serving Size: 1

Ingredients:

- 1 cup frozen peach slices

- 2 tablespoons almond butter

- 1 tablespoon honey

- 1/2 cup almond milk (unsweetened)

Instructions:

1. In a blender, combine frozen peach slices, almond butter, honey, and almond milk.

2. Blend until smooth.

3. Pour the mixture into a shallow dish and freeze for at least 4 hours.

4. Before serving, let it soften for a few minutes and scoop into a bowl.

Nutritional Information:

- Calories: 200

- Protein: 5g

- Carbohydrates: 30g

- Fat: 8g

- Fiber: 5g

7. Cinnamon Baked Pears

Prep Time: 10 minutes

Cooking Time: 30 minutes

Serving Size: 1

Ingredients:

- 2 ripe pears, halved and cored

- 1 tablespoon honey

- 1/2 teaspoon cinnamon

- 1 tablespoon chopped pecans

Instructions:

1. Preheat the oven to 375°F (190°C).

2. Place pear halves on a baking sheet.

3. Drizzle honey over each pear half.

4. Sprinkle with cinnamon and chopped pecans.

5. Bake for 30 minutes or until pears are tender.

6. Serve warm.

Nutritional Information:

- Calories: 180

- Protein: 2g

- Carbohydrates: 40g

- Fat: 5g

- Fiber: 8g

8. Blueberry and Almond Crisp

Prep Time: 15 minutes

Cooking Time: 25 minutes

Serving Size: 1

Ingredients:

- 1 cup fresh blueberries

- 1 tablespoon lemon juice

- 2 tablespoons almond flour

- 1 tablespoon honey

- 2 tablespoons rolled oats

- 1 tablespoon sliced almonds

Instructions:

1. Preheat the oven to 375°F (190°C).

2. In a bowl, toss fresh blueberries with lemon juice.

3. In a separate bowl, mix almond flour, honey, rolled oats, and sliced almonds.

4. Place blueberries in a baking dish and sprinkle the almond mixture on top.

5. Bake for 25 minutes or until the top is golden brown.

6. Serve warm.

Nutritional Information:

- Calories: 220

- Protein: 4g

- Carbohydrates: 40g

- Fat: 7g

- Fiber: 6g

9. Strawberry and Basil Sorbet

Prep Time: 10 minutes

Freezing Time: 4 hours

Serving Size: 1

Ingredients:

- 1 cup frozen strawberries

- 1 tablespoon fresh basil, chopped

- 2 tablespoons honey

- 1/2 cup water

Instructions:

1. In a blender, combine frozen strawberries, chopped fresh basil, honey, and water.

2. Blend until smooth.

3. Pour the mixture into a shallow dish and freeze for at least 4 hours.

4. Before serving, let it soften for a few minutes and scoop into a bowl.

Nutritional Information:

- Calories: 150

- Protein: 2g

- Carbohydrates: 35g

- Fat: 1g

- Fiber: 6g

10. Almond and Coconut Energy Bites

Prep Time: 15 minutes
Chilling Time: 1 hour
Serving Size: 2 bites

Ingredients:

- 1/2 cup almonds, finely chopped

- 1/4 cup unsweetened shredded coconut

- 2 tablespoons almond butter

- 2 tablespoons honey

- 1/2 teaspoon vanilla extract

Instructions:

1. In a bowl, combine chopped almonds, shredded coconut, almond butter, honey, and vanilla extract.

2. Mix until well combined.

3. Roll the mixture into small bites and place them on a plate.

4. Chill in the refrigerator for at least 1 hour before serving.

Nutritional Information:

- Calories: 180

- Protein: 5g

- Carbohydrates: 15g

- Fat: 12g

- Fiber: 3g

These dessert recipes are designed to satisfy your sweet cravings while adhering to the dietary requirements of a Stage 3 Kidney Disease diet. Enjoy these delicious and nutritious treats in moderation as part of your overall kidney-friendly meal plan. Adjust portion sizes based on your individual nutritional needs.

CHAPTER 10: 30-DAY MEAL PLAN

Day 1:

- **Breakfast:** Quinoa and Berry Breakfast Bowl

- **Lunch:** Lentil and Vegetable Soup

- **Dinner:** Chicken and Vegetable Skewers

- **Snack:** Greek Yogurt and Berry Parfait

- **Dessert:** Berry and Yogurt Parfait

Day 2:

- **Breakfast:** Spinach and Feta Omelette

- **Lunch:** Turkey and Vegetable Wrap

- **Dinner:** Lentil and Sweet Potato Curry

- **Snack:** Avocado and Tomato Salsa

- **Dessert:** Chocolate Avocado Mousse

Day 3:

- **Breakfast:** Overnight Oats with Mixed Berries

- **Lunch:** Quinoa and Black Bean Bowl

- **Dinner:** Spaghetti Squash with Tomato Sauce

- **Snack:** Cottage Cheese and Pineapple Skewers

- **Dessert:** Vanilla Chia Pudding with Fresh Mango

Day 4:

- **Breakfast:** Sweet Potato and Turkey Sausage Hash

- **Lunch:** Tuna Salad Lettuce Wraps

- **Dinner:** Grilled Vegetable and Quinoa Stuffed Bell Peppers

- **Snack:** Edamame and Sea Salt

- **Dessert:** Banana and Walnut Oat Cookies

Day 5:

- **Breakfast:** Greek Yogurt Parfait with Granola

- **Lunch:** Chickpea and Spinach Stew

- **Dinner:** Teriyaki Glazed Cod

- **Snack:** Caprese Salad Skewers

- **Dessert:** Peach and Almond Sorbet

Day 6:

- **Breakfast:** Scrambled Eggs with Spinach and Tomatoes

- **Lunch:** Shrimp and Quinoa Stir-Fry

- **Dinner:** Mediterranean Chicken and Couscous

- **Snack:** Almond Butter and Banana Slices

- **Dessert:** Cinnamon Baked Pears

Day 7:

- **Breakfast:** Banana and Walnut Pancakes

- **Lunch:** Greek Turkey Burger

- **Dinner:** Sweet Potato and Black Bean Chili

- **Snack:** Smoked Salmon and Cucumber Bites

- **Dessert:** Blueberry and Almond Crisp

Day 8:

- **Breakfast:** Avocado Toast with Poached Egg

- **Lunch:** Cauliflower Fried Rice

- **Dinner:** Pesto Zoodles with Cherry Tomatoes

- **Snack:** Quinoa and Vegetable Stuffed Mushrooms

- **Dessert:** Strawberry and Basil Sorbet

Day 9:

- **Breakfast:** Blueberry and Almond Smoothie Bowl

- **Lunch:** Quinoa Salad with Avocado and Black Beans

- **Dinner:** Chicken and Broccoli Stir-Fry

- **Snack:** Tzatziki and Whole Wheat Pita Wedges

- **Dessert:** Almond and Coconut Energy Bites

Day 10:

- **Breakfast:** Chia Seed Pudding with Mango

- **Lunch:** Lentil and Vegetable Soup

- **Dinner:** Grilled Chicken Salad with Lemon Vinaigrette

- **Snack:** Greek Yogurt and Berry Parfait

- **Dessert:** Berry and Yogurt Parfait

Day 11:

- **Breakfast:** Spinach and Feta Omelette

- **Lunch:** Turkey and Vegetable Wrap

- **Dinner:** Lentil and Sweet Potato Curry

- **Snack:** Avocado and Tomato Salsa

- **Dessert:** Chocolate Avocado Mousse

Day 12:

- **Breakfast:** Overnight Oats with Mixed Berries

- **Lunch:** Quinoa and Black Bean Bowl

- **Dinner:** Spaghetti Squash with Tomato Sauce

- **Snack:** Cottage Cheese and Pineapple Skewers

- **Dessert:** Vanilla Chia Pudding with Fresh Mango

Day 13:

- **Breakfast:** Sweet Potato and Turkey Sausage Hash

- **Lunch:** Tuna Salad Lettuce Wraps

- **Dinner:** Grilled Vegetable and Quinoa Stuffed Bell Peppers

- **Snack:** Edamame and Sea Salt

- **Dessert:** Banana and Walnut Oat Cookies

Day 14:

- **Breakfast:** Greek Yogurt Parfait with Granola

- **Lunch:** Chickpea and Spinach Stew

- **Dinner:** Teriyaki Glazed Cod

- **Snack:** Caprese Salad Skewers

- **Dessert:** Peach and Almond Sorbet

Day 15:

- **Breakfast:** Scrambled Eggs with Spinach and Tomatoes

- **Lunch:** Shrimp and Quinoa Stir-Fry

- **Dinner:** Mediterranean Chicken and Couscous

- **Snack:** Almond Butter and Banana Slices

- **Dessert:** Cinnamon Baked Pears

Day 16:

- **Breakfast:** Banana and Walnut Pancakes

- **Lunch:** Greek Turkey Burger

- **Dinner:** Sweet Potato and Black Bean Chili

- **Snack:** Smoked Salmon and Cucumber Bites

- **Dessert:** Blueberry and Almond Crisp

Day 17:

- **Breakfast:** Avocado Toast with Poached Egg

- **Lunch:** Cauliflower Fried Rice

- **Dinner:** Pesto Zoodles with Cherry Tomatoes

- **Snack:** Quinoa and Vegetable Stuffed Mushrooms

- **Dessert:** Strawberry and Basil Sorbet

Day 18:

- **Breakfast:** Blueberry and Almond Smoothie Bowl

- **Lunch:** Quinoa Salad with Avocado and Black Beans

- **Dinner:** Chicken and Broccoli Stir-Fry

- **Snack:** Tzatziki and Whole Wheat Pita Wedges

- **Dessert:** Almond and Coconut Energy Bites

Day 19:

- **Breakfast:** Chia Seed Pudding with Mango

- **Lunch:** Lentil and Vegetable Soup

- **Dinner:** Grilled Chicken Salad with Lemon Vinaigrette

- **Snack:** Greek Yogurt and Berry Parfait

- **Dessert:** Berry and Yogurt Parfait

Day 20:

- **Breakfast:** Spinach and Feta Omelette

- **Lunch:** Turkey and Vegetable Wrap

- **Dinner:** Lentil and Sweet Potato Curry

- **Snack:** Avocado and Tomato Salsa

- **Dessert:** Chocolate Avocado Mousse

Day 21:

- **Breakfast:** Overnight Oats with Mixed Berries

- **Lunch:** Quinoa and Black Bean Bowl

- **Dinner:** Spaghetti Squash with Tomato Sauce

- **Snack:** Cottage Cheese and Pineapple Skewers

- **Dessert:** Vanilla Chia Pudding with Fresh Mango

Day 22:

- **Breakfast:** Sweet Potato and Turkey Sausage Hash

- **Lunch:** Tuna Salad Lettuce Wraps

- **Dinner:** Grilled Vegetable and Quinoa Stuffed Bell Peppers

- **Snack:** Edamame and Sea Salt

- **Dessert:** Banana and Walnut Oat Cookies

Day 23:

- **Breakfast:** Greek Yogurt Parfait with Granola

- **Lunch:** Chickpea and Spinach Stew

- **Dinner:** Teriyaki Glazed Cod

- **Snack:** Caprese Salad Skewers

- **Dessert:** Peach and Almond Sorbet

Day 24:

- **Breakfast:** Scrambled Eggs with Spinach and Tomatoes

- **Lunch:** Shrimp and Quinoa Stir-Fry

- **Dinner:** Mediterranean Chicken and Couscous

- **Snack:** Almond Butter and Banana Slices

- **Dessert:** Cinnamon Baked Pears

Day 25:

- **Breakfast:** Banana and Walnut Pancakes

- **Lunch:** Greek Turkey Burger

- **Dinner:** Sweet Potato and Black Bean Chili

- **Snack:** Smoked Salmon and Cucumber Bites

- **Dessert:** Blueberry and Almond Crisp

Day 26:

- **Breakfast:** Avocado Toast with Poached Egg

- **Lunch:** Cauliflower Fried Rice

- **Dinner:** Pesto Zoodles with Cherry Tomatoes

- **Snack:** Quinoa and Vegetable Stuffed Mushrooms

- **Dessert:** Strawberry and Basil Sorbet

Day 27:

- **Breakfast:** Blueberry and Almond Smoothie Bowl

- **Lunch:** Quinoa Salad with Avocado and Black Beans

- **Dinner:** Chicken and Broccoli Stir-Fry

- **Snack:** Tzatziki and Whole Wheat Pita Wedges

- **Dessert:** Almond and Coconut Energy Bites

Day 28:

- **Breakfast:** Chia Seed Pudding with Mango

- **Lunch:** Lentil and Vegetable Soup

- **Dinner:** Grilled Chicken Salad with Lemon Vinaigrette

- **Snack:** Greek Yogurt and Berry Parfait

- **Dessert:** Berry and Yogurt Parfait

Day 29:

- **Breakfast:** Spinach and Feta Omelette

- **Lunch:** Turkey and Vegetable Wrap

- **Dinner:** Lentil and Sweet Potato Curry

- **Snack:** Avocado and Tomato Salsa

- **Dessert:** Chocolate Avocado Mousse

Day 30:

- **Breakfast:** Overnight Oats with Mixed Berries

- **Lunch:** Quinoa and Black Bean Bowl

- **Dinner:** Spaghetti Squash with Tomato Sauce

- **Snack:** Cottage Cheese and Pineapple Skewers

- **Dessert:** Vanilla Chia Pudding with Fresh Mango

CHAPTER 11: LIFESTYLE CHANGES FOR KIDNEY HEALTH

The journey toward optimal kidney health involves more than just dietary adjustments. While a kidney-friendly diet is crucial, incorporating lifestyle changes is equally significant for comprehensive well-being. In this chapter, we delve into three pivotal aspects of lifestyle changes: Exercise and Physical Activity, Stress Management, and the Importance of Adequate Sleep.

Exercise and Physical Activity

Embracing an active lifestyle is a cornerstone of maintaining kidney health. Engaging in regular exercise not only contributes to overall physical well-being but also plays a key role in supporting kidney function. The benefits of exercise extend beyond the cardiovascular system, positively impacting various facets of health.

When it comes to kidney health, regular physical activity aids in maintaining a healthy blood pressure, a critical factor in preventing kidney damage. High blood pressure is a leading cause of kidney disease, and exercise acts as a natural mechanism to regulate blood pressure levels. It enhances the efficiency of the cardiovascular system, reducing the strain on the kidneys.

Moreover, exercise promotes weight management, another essential element for kidney health. Obesity is a risk factor for kidney disease, and incorporating physical activity into one's routine helps in achieving and maintaining a healthy weight. This is particularly significant for individuals with kidney concerns, as excess weight can exacerbate existing conditions.

A variety of exercises can be beneficial for kidney health. Cardiovascular exercises like walking, jogging, or cycling enhance heart function and improve blood circulation, benefiting the kidneys. Strength training exercises, such as weightlifting or resistance training, contribute to overall muscle health and metabolism, indirectly supporting kidney function.

It's important to note that the intensity and duration of exercise should be tailored to individual fitness levels and health conditions. Consulting with a healthcare professional before starting an exercise regimen, especially for those with pre-existing kidney conditions, ensures a safe and effective approach to physical activity.

Incorporating exercise into a daily routine doesn't necessarily require a gym membership or specialized equipment. Simple activities like brisk walking, gardening, or taking the stairs can contribute significantly to overall physical well-being. The key is consistency – making physical activity a regular part of life.

In summary, exercise and physical activity are integral components of a holistic approach to kidney health. Regular, moderate exercise not only supports cardiovascular health and weight management but also plays a crucial role in maintaining optimal kidney function.

Stress Management

Chronic stress has been recognized as a potential contributor to various health issues, including kidney disease. Understanding and managing stress are essential aspects of promoting overall well-being and supporting kidney health.

The body's response to stress involves the release of hormones like cortisol and adrenaline, which can impact blood pressure and heart rate. Prolonged or chronic stress can contribute to hypertension, a significant risk factor for kidney disease. Therefore, incorporating effective stress management techniques is crucial for individuals aiming to protect their kidneys.

One effective method of stress management is adopting relaxation techniques. Practices such as deep breathing, meditation, and yoga have been shown to reduce stress levels and promote a sense of calm. These techniques not only have a direct impact on stress but also contribute to overall mental and emotional well-being.

Another important aspect of stress management is identifying and addressing the sources of stress in one's life. This may involve making lifestyle changes, setting realistic goals, and learning to prioritize tasks. Seeking support from friends, family, or a mental health professional can be instrumental in navigating stressors and developing coping strategies.

Physical activity, which we discussed in the previous section, also plays a role in stress management. Exercise releases endorphins, often referred to as "feel-good" hormones, which can elevate mood and alleviate stress. Engaging in regular physical activity, even in moderate amounts, can contribute significantly to stress reduction.

Creating a supportive environment is key to effective stress management. This includes fostering positive relationships, maintaining a healthy work-life balance, and cultivating hobbies and activities that bring joy and relaxation. Establishing boundaries and learning to say no when necessary are important components of creating a stress-resilient lifestyle.

In conclusion, stress management is a vital aspect of kidney health. By adopting relaxation techniques, addressing the sources of stress, and incorporating physical activity, individuals can reduce the impact of chronic stress on their overall well-being and support optimal kidney function.

Importance of Adequate Sleep

Sleep is a fundamental pillar of overall health, and its significance extends to kidney health. Adequate and quality sleep plays a crucial role in various physiological processes, including kidney function and repair.

During sleep, the body undergoes a series of essential processes, such as tissue repair, hormone regulation, and immune system strengthening. These processes are integral to maintaining optimal health, and any disruption in sleep patterns can impact these functions.

One of the key connections between sleep and kidney health is the regulation of blood pressure. Sleep deprivation or poor sleep quality can lead to an increase in blood pressure, placing additional strain on the kidneys. Over time, this elevated blood pressure can contribute to the development or progression of kidney disease.

Moreover, sleep influences the body's hormonal balance, including hormones related to stress and metabolism. Disruptions in sleep patterns can lead to imbalances in cortisol, insulin, and other hormones, potentially contributing to metabolic issues and inflammation, both of which can affect kidney health.

For individuals with existing kidney conditions, prioritizing adequate sleep is especially important. Chronic kidney disease is associated with an increased risk of sleep disturbances, creating a potential cycle where compromised sleep further impacts kidney function.

Establishing healthy sleep hygiene practices is essential for promoting restful and restorative sleep. This includes maintaining a consistent sleep schedule, creating a comfortable sleep environment, and avoiding stimulants like caffeine close to bedtime. Additionally, limiting screen time before sleep and practicing relaxation techniques can contribute to improved sleep quality.

In cases where sleep disturbances persist, consulting with a healthcare professional is advisable. Identifying and addressing potential sleep disorders or underlying health issues can contribute to better sleep outcomes and, consequently, improved kidney health.

CHAPTER 12: MONITORING AND ADJUSTING THE DIET PLAN

Embarking on a kidney disease diet is a proactive step toward managing and improving kidney health. However, the journey doesn't end with the initial dietary changes. Regular monitoring, awareness of warning signs, and making necessary adjustments to the diet plan are crucial elements for long-term kidney health. In this chapter, we explore these aspects in detail.

Regular Check-ups and Lab Tests

Regular check-ups and laboratory tests are fundamental components of kidney health maintenance. These assessments provide valuable insights into the functioning of the kidneys and help healthcare professionals monitor any changes or potential issues. Incorporating these check-ups into your routine is essential for staying proactive about your kidney health.

For individuals with kidney disease, healthcare providers typically recommend regular monitoring through blood tests and urine tests. These tests assess key indicators of kidney function, including serum creatinine levels, glomerular filtration rate (GFR), and the presence of protein or other abnormalities in the urine.

Serum creatinine is a waste product produced by muscle metabolism and excreted by the kidneys. Elevated levels may indicate impaired kidney function. GFR is a measure of how efficiently the kidneys filter waste from the blood. A decline in GFR may suggest a decrease in kidney function. Proteinuria, the presence of excess protein in the urine, can be a sign of kidney damage.

The frequency of these tests depends on the severity of kidney disease and the individual's overall health. For those with more advanced kidney disease, more frequent monitoring may be necessary. It's crucial to follow the healthcare provider's recommendations regarding the timing of these tests.

Regular check-ups also allow healthcare professionals to assess and manage other factors that can impact kidney health, such as blood pressure, blood sugar levels, and medications. High blood pressure and uncontrolled diabetes are risk factors for kidney disease, and managing these conditions is integral to kidney health.

Participating actively in your healthcare journey includes keeping track of your test results, understanding the implications, and discussing any concerns or questions with your healthcare team. Open communication ensures that adjustments to the treatment plan, including dietary recommendations, can be made promptly based on your individual health status.

Recognizing Warning Signs

While regular check-ups and lab tests provide objective data about kidney function, recognizing warning signs and symptoms is equally important. Being attuned to changes in your body and addressing potential issues early can prevent complications and support better kidney health.

Some common warning signs of kidney issues include changes in urinary patterns, swelling in the legs or face, persistent fatigue, and unexplained weight loss. Changes in urine color, frequency, or the presence of foamy urine may indicate underlying kidney concerns. Swelling, particularly in the extremities, can be a sign of fluid retention, which may be related to impaired kidney function.

Persistent fatigue and unexplained weight loss can also signal potential kidney issues. The kidneys play a crucial role in producing erythropoietin, a hormone that stimulates red blood cell production. Impaired kidney function can lead to anemia, contributing to fatigue. Unintended weight loss may be associated with changes in appetite or metabolic imbalances.

It's important to note that these symptoms are nonspecific and can be indicative of various health conditions. However, if you experience any of these warning signs, it's essential to consult with your healthcare provider promptly. Early intervention and appropriate management can prevent further progression of kidney disease and improve overall health outcomes.

In addition to physical symptoms, individuals with kidney concerns should be mindful of their mental and emotional well-being. Chronic kidney disease is associated with an increased risk of depression and anxiety. Recognizing changes in mood, sleep patterns, or coping mechanisms is essential for holistic health management.

Taking a proactive approach to recognizing warning signs involves self-awareness, regular self-checks, and open communication with healthcare providers. Regular dialogue with your healthcare team ensures that any emerging issues can be addressed promptly, facilitating timely adjustments to the treatment plan.

Making Adjustments to the Diet

Dietary adjustments play a central role in managing kidney disease, and making timely modifications to the diet plan is a dynamic aspect of kidney health maintenance. As kidney function evolves or changes, adapting the diet to meet specific needs is crucial for optimal well-being.

The dietary recommendations for kidney health are not static; they may need to be modified based on factors such as the progression of kidney disease, changes in overall health, or the presence of comorbidities. Regular monitoring of kidney function through lab tests provides the necessary data to guide these adjustments.

In the early stages of kidney disease, dietary modifications often focus on reducing sodium, phosphorus, and potassium intake.

Controlling protein intake may also be a consideration, depending on individual health status. As kidney disease progresses, the dietary approach may need to be more restrictive to manage complications and maintain balance.

For individuals on a kidney disease diet, it's essential to work closely with a registered dietitian or healthcare professional. These professionals can provide personalized guidance based on lab results, dietary preferences, and lifestyle factors. Regular follow-up appointments allow for ongoing assessment and adjustments to the diet plan as needed.

One common adjustment in a kidney disease diet is managing fluid intake. As kidney function declines, the ability to regulate fluid balance may be compromised. Monitoring daily fluid intake becomes crucial, and adjustments may be necessary based on individual needs. It's important to strike a balance between staying adequately hydrated and avoiding excessive fluid retention.

Phosphorus management is another critical aspect of dietary adjustments. High phosphorus levels in the blood can contribute to bone and cardiovascular issues in individuals with kidney disease. Limiting phosphorus-rich foods, including certain dairy products and processed foods, may be necessary.

Potassium control is particularly important for those with compromised kidney function. Abnormal potassium levels can impact heart health. Foods high in potassium, such as bananas, oranges, and potatoes, may need to be limited or carefully monitored.

Protein intake is a nuanced aspect of dietary adjustments. While protein is essential for overall health, excessive protein intake can burden the kidneys. Adjusting protein levels based on individual requirements and health status is an ongoing consideration in managing kidney disease.

CONCLUSION

And there you have it – the comprehensive journey through the pages of "Kidney Disease Diet for Stage 3." As we close this book, it's not just about reaching the last page; it's about embracing a roadmap for kidney health that extends far beyond the final chapter.

Our exploration started with a deep dive into understanding Stage 3 Kidney Disease, unraveling its nuances, and demystifying the stages that precede it. We uncovered the importance of a kidney-friendly diet, not as a restrictive set of rules but as a vibrant palette of nourishment tailored to support and heal.

Chapter by chapter, we traversed the landscape of kidney health, each section revealing its unique facets. We learned about the vital nutrients, delved into the intricacies of sodium, potassium, and phosphorus, and mastered the art of crafting a kidney-friendly diet plan. From deciphering food labels to savoring kidney-friendly recipes, the culinary journey became a celebration of both health and flavor.

But this book is more than just a collection of facts and guidelines; it's a companion on your quest for well-being. The lifestyle changes we explored – from the importance of exercise and stress management to the often-underestimated value of a good night's sleep – are not just recommendations but invitations to embrace a holistic approach to health.

Regular check-ups and lab tests became your checkpoints, providing insights into the intricate dance of your kidneys. Recognizing warning signs became an empowering skill, an acknowledgment that your body communicates, and listening can be a transformative act. And in the midst of it all, the flexibility to make adjustments to your diet plan emerged as the secret ingredient – a reminder that health is dynamic, and so should be our responses to it.

As we part ways, remember this: every choice you make, every meal you savor, and every step you take contributes to the narrative of your kidney health. It's a journey marked by progress, not perfection. There might be twists and turns, but armed with knowledge and a dash of adaptability, you have the tools to navigate them all.

Take the essence of this book with you – the flavors of kidney-friendly recipes, the wisdom of lifestyle changes, and the empowerment to actively participate in your well-being. Let it be your guide as you continue to nourish your kidneys and, in turn, yourself.

So here's to your health – to vibrant mornings, energized afternoons, and restful nights. May your kidneys thrive, your body flourish, and your spirit embrace the richness of a life well-lived. Until we meet again on the journey to optimal well-being, stay healthy, stay vibrant, and savor every chapter of your life.

9 798877 929500